Essential Clinical Social Work Series

Series Editor
Carol Tosone, School of Social Work, New York University, New York, NY, USA

More information about this series at http://www.springer.com/series/8115

John P. McTighe

Narrative Theory in Clinical Social Work Practice

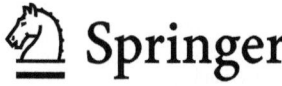
Springer

John P. McTighe
School of Social Science and Human Services
Ramapo College
Mahwah, NJ, USA

ISSN 2520-1611   ISSN 2520-162X (electronic)
Essential Clinical Social Work Series
ISBN 978-3-319-70786-0   ISBN 978-3-319-70787-7 (eBook)
https://doi.org/10.1007/978-3-319-70787-7

Library of Congress Control Number: 2017962420

© Springer International Publishing AG 2018
This work is subject to copyright. All rights are reserved by the Publisher, whether the whole or part of the material is concerned, specifically the rights of translation, reprinting, reuse of illustrations, recitation, broadcasting, reproduction on microfilms or in any other physical way, and transmission or information storage and retrieval, electronic adaptation, computer software, or by similar or dissimilar methodology now known or hereafter developed.
The use of general descriptive names, registered names, trademarks, service marks, etc. in this publication does not imply, even in the absence of a specific statement, that such names are exempt from the relevant protective laws and regulations and therefore free for general use.
The publisher, the authors and the editors are safe to assume that the advice and information in this book are believed to be true and accurate at the date of publication. Neither the publisher nor the authors or the editors give a warranty, express or implied, with respect to the material contained herein or for any errors or omissions that may have been made. The publisher remains neutral with regard to jurisdictional claims in published maps and institutional affiliations.

Printed on acid-free paper

This Springer imprint is published by Springer Nature
The registered company is Springer International Publishing AG
The registered company address is: Gewerbestrasse 11, 6330 Cham, Switzerland

For Ivannia,
The heart of my story

Preface

I am a storyteller. Over the years I have wrestled a bit with this aspect of myself. After all, I am an academic, a professor. But if you ask anyone who knows me—my wife and children, friends, extended family, colleagues, and yes, perhaps especially my students—those sometimes involuntary recipients of my tales—I suspect they will agree. I tell stories.

However, I've realized over the years, whether in my personal life or my professional life, that I don't just tell stories because I think this or that one is interesting or funny or heartwarming. I do it because I believe that stories really are the stuff of life; they are the framework that holds together our sense of self and the world—the way we make meaning. They are the way we connect with others. To my way of thinking, stories help us take all that we know—all that information that we may have voraciously or may be reluctantly consumed—and put it into action.

When I was in Social Work School, I had the opportunity to take an excellent course on Object Relations Theory. It was a hugely popular class, mostly because of the person who taught it. We read everyone from Freud to Kernberg. If you know anything about Object Relations (though that isn't necessary in order to follow *this* story), you understand that the work of its theorists can be dense and heady; they sometimes seem like they are speaking a foreign language. What I noticed among my classmates was that, after a short time, the goal of that course for many of them was getting through as painlessly as possible to graduation. But for me, Object Relations meant something different. For me it was as though someone had thrown a light on and showed me a way of understanding people that I had never contemplated before.

Now I will admit that I am a very abstract thinker, and that comes with its upsides and downsides (e.g., I can't understand how a computer works to save my life and I wouldn't even attempt to do my own taxes). So I did enjoy learning the concepts and lexicon of Object Relations quite a bit. But I realized that more than anything what made it accessible and even useful to me was what I was able to hear in all that abstract complexity—stories. The readings and concepts offered me a way into the stories of the clients I was working with, a way of understanding their pain, the roots of their fragility, and the way the world looked to them because of their stories. But the theory did something else as well. It offered a lens through which to envision new narrative possibilities—ways of continuing the creation of those stories along lines that were more healing and more filled with hope.

So for me, this is a good deal of what narrative is about in the context of a book like the one you are holding in your hands. It is the same thing that I hope narrative (*story*) is about for the students who sit in my classroom. Stories are a way in. They are a way of seeing, feeling, and connecting with ourselves and those around us. In the context of the clinical situation, they are a bridge—a bridge into the internal world of the client, as well as a bridge between them and us and the social environment. These stories include the ones they have crafted about themselves, life and the world, as well as the ones that are being co-constructed by them and us as we sit together in the uniquely intimate expanse and containment of a therapeutic space.

One of my children was asking the other day at the dinner table about the first foods she ate as a baby. She was born in the beginning of August, and if you have any experience with the care and feeding of newborns, you know that it takes a few months before they can digest solid food. So we recalled with a laugh a great photo from her first Thanksgiving, when she was a little more than 3 months old. She is sitting on my wife's lap, proudly sporting her turkey bib, enormous drumstick in hand, looking adorably bewildered. It was time for her first solid food. In point of fact, we told her, her meal that day was a thin combination of breast milk and rice cereal. Happy Thanksgiving!

Believe it or not, this story does have bearing on the matter at hand. All teachers know that facilitating a learning experience for students is not simply a matter of offering up mountains of information. I believe that what leads to learning is making all of that information digestible. Please don't be mistaken by the baby metaphor. There is nothing in what I am saying here that is intended to be paternalistic or patronizing. But I think that we all need a way of digesting information in a manner that will help us make use of it. For me, stories facilitate that; they always have.

As we travel together through this book then, here is what I am proposing. I will offer you a lot of information—theory, research, and clinical application. And I will tell you a lot of stories. My hope is that the stories will put flesh on the bones of the rest and help you digest it, hold on to it, and make it useful for yourself and your clients. I am not proposing to offer you here a cookbook of narrative recipes or techniques. Instead, what I hope to offer is something that I firmly believe will be more useful for you in the long run—and that is a way of listening, thinking, engaging, and working.

Mahwah, NJ, USA   John P. McTighe

Acknowledgements

There are many people to whom I owe a debt of gratitude for their assistance and support as I worked on this book. Carol Tosone, the Editor of the Essential Clinical Social Work Series, has been a wonderful mentor and friend for nearly 15 years. From the days when she chaired my dissertation committee to her ongoing encouragement and belief in my work, she has been exceedingly generous in her support and I could not be more grateful to her. I would also like to thank Jennifer Hadley and the editorial staff at Springer for their support in the completion of this project.

Ramapo College of New Jersey has become a wonderful academic home to me. It is an increasingly rare thing in the academic world today to find a place where one truly has the freedom to pursue scholarly passions and ideas. Ramapo is such a place, and I am grateful to be there. Dean Aaron R.S. Lorenz of the School of Social Science and Human Services, Assistant Dean for Social Work Ann Marie Moreno, and all my colleagues in the Social Work Convening Group are an outstanding source of support and collegiality, and it is an honor to work with them. I offer thanks to my students, whose passion and commitment remind me continually of all I love about the profession of social work. It is a joy to teach them.

My deepest expression of gratitude goes to the clients who have allowed me to accompany them for a time and who have invited me into some of the most sacred places in their lives, especially those whose stories appear in some form in this book. It is a privilege to be a part of their journey.

And to my family… The enthusiasm and encouragement of my daughters, Hannah and Sarah, mean more to me than I can say. As I write this, I am looking at the white board that hangs on the wall above my desk. It is covered by their messages, left as surprises, assurances of their love and their confidence in me. My wife, Ivannia, to whom I have dedicated this book, is my muse and my great love. Her patience and support are unparalleled. Her belief in me is unwavering. I could never have done this without her.

About the Author

John P. McTighe is currently an Assistant Professor of Social Work at Ramapo College of New Jersey. He received his master's degree in social work and Ph.D. in clinical social work from the Silver School of Social Work at New York University, and his M.Div. from the Washington Theological Union in Silver Spring, Maryland. He has published numerous articles in journals such as *British Journal of Social Work*, *Journal of Traumatic Stress*, and *Clinical Social Work Journal*, in addition to contributing a chapter to *Critical Thinking in Clinical Assessment and Diagnosis*. He is also in private practice in Pompton Plains, New Jersey.

Contents

1 Narrative Theory: An Introduction and Overview 1
2 Encountering the Self, Encountering the Other: Narratives of Race and Ethnicity 19
3 Surviving Together: Individual and Communal Narratives in the Wake of Tragedy...................................... 43
4 Spiritual Stories: Exploring Ultimate Meaning in Social Work Practice 67
5 Sexual Stories: Narratives of Sexual Identity, Gender, and Sexual Development 85
6 Leaving Home, Finding Home: Narrative Practice with Immigrant Populations....................................... 113
7 Moving on: Narrative Perspectives on Grief and Loss 143
8 Who I Am and Who I Want to Be: Narrative and the Evolving Self of the Social Worker in Clinical Practice 171

Index.. 183

Introduction

Social workers, and in fact all clinicians, are continually searching for ways to engage clients, and to help them grow in their understanding of themselves and the meaning of their experience. In this way, we strive to help our clients find healing, growth, and deeper satisfaction in their daily living. As a professor and a practicing social worker, however, I know how overwhelming it can be to try to make sense of the seemingly endless complexities of theory and practice, and particularly the relationship between the two. It is a conversation that I have with my students all the time.

In this book, I will present what is both a theoretical point of view and an approach to practice—Narrative. My hope is that I will do so in a manner that helps you make sense of not only the theoretical underpinnings of narrative, but also the way in which it can be applied to a variety of situations and concerns that social workers and other clinicians routinely encounter.

The first supervisor I ever had as a social work student commented once that there was a pattern or habit she noticed in my process recordings that she didn't particularly like. When I was listening to clients or gathering the details of something that had happened to them, it seems I would fairly often ask, "What was that like for you?" My supervisor suggested that I stop asking it because she said it wasn't a very helpful question. What was the point of it? What information of value did it yield? I took her question thoughtfully of course. I really did. I was (and still am) eager to be a good interviewer and a skilled diagnostician and clinician. Just as you'd expect following a good supervisory moment, I actually began to notice myself asking that question. It came from me quite naturally—without any forethought.

So why was I asking it? "What was that like for you?" I had been interested in and did work on narrative before I went to social work school. I had even written a previous master's thesis on it. But I didn't piece together until then, that narrative was the springboard for that questionable question. Though I am certain that I took my supervisor's comments to heart and started to use the question more thoughtfully and even sparingly, I know I didn't abandon it altogether. In a way I couldn't have articulated at the time as a beginning clinician, I really believed in and sensed the value of tuning in to the depth of a person's story—listening to them and wondering about *the more*... How did they experience this or that event or part of their history?

What meaning did they make of it? I wanted to communicate a deep interest in their experience—an experience that I noticed often enough they themselves hadn't been able to reflect on all that carefully.

One of the challenges faced by beginning and even many seasoned social workers is the lack of a theoretical base that grounds the way they think and work. If they are not able to grasp theory and understand how it relates to practice, many are left floundering in the consulting room. When paired with the anxiety that leads many beginning clinicians to seek out and rely on a "toolkit" of techniques and strategies they can call on in a pinch, this can lead to a clinical approach that lacks depth and coherence.

I recall once asking a senior and seasoned social worker what it meant when clinicians said they were "eclectic." She responded that there are social workers who, by virtue of their knowledge base and experience, are able to weave together the insights and strategies of varied perspectives as they listen, much like a chef who knows intuitively which ingredients will best complement each other. For many though, the term "eclectic" suggested something far less artful or purposeful. It suggested a lack of grounding. "In order to be eclectic," she said, "you have to have a point of view."

My hope in this book is to introduce social work students and other interested readers to a particular way of listening, thinking, and working. Though many social workers may hear the term narrative in the course of their education, they are not commonly introduced to the fullness of narrative theory and the implications it has for the practice of clinical social work. For this reason, *Narrative Theory in Clinical Social Work Practice* will begin with a discussion of the history and current state of narrative theory and what I believe it has to offer to the contemporary practice of clinical social work. Subsequent chapters will then go on to address the implications of narrative for an understanding of race and ethnicity, trauma, spirituality, and sexuality. We will also examine the implications of narrative theory for practice with immigrant populations and in the area of grief and loss. Finally, we will consider the meaning of narrative for the development of the professional self of the clinician. Each chapter will speak to the way narrative theory informs the work of listening and intervening in the clinical situation. Furthermore, written with you, the social work student, in mind, the book as a whole will be formatted to facilitate its use in the educational setting. Every chapter begins with a series of guiding questions and keywords meant to orient you to the substance of the chapter, and ends with questions and activities for further reflection. These may be used on your own, to deepen your learning, or by your instructor, as a component of a social work course.

My plan is to write as if we were together in the classroom. I will pose questions to you, the reader. At times I may ask you to tune into your own reactions to what I have written, or to engage your own stories as well as your imagination. Not surprisingly I suppose, when I teach I often use stories, and I will share quite a few here. Because, as we will explore throughout the book, our narratives are rarely if ever about *one* thing, you will notice that the themes in the stories I tell are overlapping, likely touching on the subject area of more than one chapter. This is natural and to be expected. Please know that, in the interest of confidentiality and the protection of clients' privacy, I have modified the clinical narratives that I use throughout this book, changing names, places, and in some instances other details of their stories, without altering the points that the cases are meant to convey. I hope these illustrations put some meat on the bones, as it were, and help make the information I am offering you both digestible and something you can hold onto and make use of.

A word about terminology… Throughout the book, I will vary the term I use for the person in the role of the helping professional. Sometimes I will refer to the social worker. At other times I will speak of the clinician, or the therapist. People refer to themselves professionally by any number of designations, and not all of them may feel like they "fit," or represent the particular kind of professional you are striving to become. That, in fact, has to do with your own personal narrative. Not all social workers identify as clinicians or therapists. Nor should they. However, for the purposes of this book, I will treat the terms as more or less interchangeable. Similarly, while the books in the *Essential Clinical Social Work* series are particularly aimed at social work students, it is my intention and hope that this book will be equally as useful for more seasoned practitioners who are interested in learning about narrative, as well as for students of other professions such as psychology, psychiatry, counseling, pastoral counseling, and marriage and family therapy.

So if you're ready, let's begin!

Chapter 1
Narrative Theory: An Introduction and Overview

Guiding Questions

What do we mean by narrative and what are its implications for the practice of clinical social work?

What are the philosophical underpinnings of narrative theory and what do they have to tell us about the human person and our quest for identity and meaning?

What is the relationship between the narratives we construct and what we generally think of as "truth"?

What are the key dimensions of our presence with clients as social workers working from a narrative perspective?

How are we to understand the reflexive relationship between narrative and culture?

Some time ago, as I was walking across campus with a colleague, she ran into a young man who had graduated from our program the year before I joined the faculty. She was clearly happy to see him, and I quickly understood that he had been an excellent student. As she introduced us she told the young man, "This is Dr. McTighe. You should really talk to him. He studies narrative." "Really?" the young man asked. "Yes," I replied. "Are you interested in narrative?" He pondered that for a moment and said, "It depends. What do you mean by narrative?" My eyes widened a bit and I told him, "Well, that's exactly the right question to ask!" Whether he knew it or not, that young student was articulating a question that scholars have been pondering and debating for decades: What is narrative?

This is a book about narrative and its role in the theory and practice of clinical social work. Through each chapter we will consider the contribution of the narrative perspective to a variety of contexts and with a variety of client populations. As we take this journey, it is my hope that we will come to a clearer understanding of narrative and the ways in which it can enhance our thinking and our practice. But in order to have some solid ground on which to stand, it is important that we lay a foundation—a clear sense of what we mean when we talk about narrative.

The first time I went to a conference on narrative to present a paper I had been working on, I felt like a fish out of water. I was the only social worker there, at least as far as I could tell. To my surprise honestly, I was surrounded instead by literature professors, philosophers, anthropologists, and historians. At times, it felt as though we were speaking different languages. We thought of narrative in seemingly different terms, cited different theorists, and saw different implications to our work. What that conference taught me, among other things, was just how diverse the world of narrative is. And, as is often the case, listening to and reflecting on multiple points of view did a great deal to clarify and even enhance my own thinking.

Like all stories based on living human experience, the story of narrative is an ever-evolving one. And like all stories of human experience, the perspective or interpretation you get will depend on the person you ask. Literary theorists, anthropologists, historians, philosophers, psychologists, and social workers understand and apply the narrative perspective each through their own lens and from their own vantage point. As interest in narrative has proliferated over the past 30–40 years, some have even posed the question of whether narrative has come to mean "anything and everything" (Riessman & Quinney, 2005, p. 393). That said, while our understanding of narrative may be very broad, we will nonetheless attempt to sketch an outline of what narrative is. In this chapter, we consider an overview of narrative theory and some of its philosophical underpinnings. Flowing from this, we will look at the way narrative has had an impact on the humanities and the social sciences broadly speaking. We then take a look at the meaning and applications of narrative for the practice of social work in a general sense.

The Conceptual History of Narrative

Though a full exploration of the conceptual history of narrative is beyond the scope of this chapter, it is nonetheless important for us to take a tour through it to understand the state of the debate and have a clearer sense of the perspective that social work can bring to bear on the theory of narrative and its implications for clinical practice.

In the 1960s, a shift began to occur, first in the field of literary criticism, then history, and later (more into the 1980s) in the social sciences. This shift has been called the "narrative turn," or inasmuch as it has presented itself differently in diverse fields of inquiry, "narrative turns" (Hyvarinen, 2010). At its root, the narrative turn emerged from movements within the philosophical landscape that began to reconsider the nature of knowledge and what we consensually refer to as "reality." What are we able to know? How? And with what degree of certainty?

Narrative falls under the broad umbrella of a school of thought known as *postmodernism*. Its philosophical predecessors, *modernism* or some might say *positivism*, were deeply invested in the human capacity to achieve knowledge and understanding through reason. Modernism espoused a view of reality, nature, etc. as inherently and objectively knowable in and of itself, particularly through the application of human reason. By contrast, postmodernism takes a skeptical view of this stance and suggests that while the world is of course *real*, our access to it through knowledge and understanding is contingent, hampered by the limitations of time and the culture-bound men and women who observe and comment on reality.

Consider for example that, centuries ago, reasonable people held with great certainty that the world is flat and pointed to all the reliable scientific evidence that this was the case. As an epistemological stance, postmodern thinking suggests that our ability to know is impacted by the inherent biases that each of us brings to the task of observation, thought, and reflection as *knowers*. In other words, what I know is conditioned on who I am as a knower. If you have had the opportunity to travel to a different part of the world, or even to spend some time immersed in a culture that is very different from your own, you likely already have an intuitive sense of what this is all about. Two human beings observing a phenomenon from radically different points of view may in fact see quite different things and have very distinct thoughts and feelings about it. What is more, they may have entirely different systems of language that they use to express those points of view and the meaning they make out of what they experience (Freedman & Combs, 1996).

Under this broad umbrella of postmodern thought, we must consider a related perspective: social constructionism. As one dimension of the postmodern point of view, social constructionism takes the view that not only is the knowability of the world and our actual knowledge of it limited by our own perspective, but also this perspective is constructed by the social and cultural environment in which we develop (Gergen, 2015). None of us exists in a vacuum. Social constructionism holds that we are each shaped by the perhaps countless subtle dimensions of the social world in which we live, and that we individually and collectively take part in the ongoing creation of that world and the meaning we make of it. In other words, our environment shapes us and we in turn shape our environment. This has enormous implications for, and gives rise to, the narrative perspective that is the heart of our consideration here. It is also worth noting that this understanding is particularly important to a narrative approach to clinical social work given the biopsychosociospiritual perspective that fundamentally undergirds our work. Emerging from this social constructionist perspective, narrative theory in its simplest iteration looks at the way human beings recount their experience of being human and give meaning to that experience. For our purposes as clinical social workers, this has significant implications for our understanding of people and practice.

As a critique of culture and the many ways of knowing, postmodernism and social constructionism alert us to the ways in which cultures and societies, as well as the many subgroups of which they are composed, commonly seek to reify their perspective or their "knowledge" as if it is inherently true and immutable for all people at all times and in all places—as if it exists "out there" in a purely discoverable way (Neimeyer, 1993). In short, they believe they have a lock on truth. This phenomenon is played out on every level from the individual to the family, group, organization, and community. We see it displayed in media, popular culture, music, and political campaigns and international relations. It comes to us in the form of extended debates and arguments, as well as slogans, bumper stickers, and social media messages. If we listen carefully, we are surrounded by messages seeking to convince us of the "truth," of the way things *really* are.

Berger and Luckmann (1966) in their seminal writing on social construction suggest that this process of reification has several components, namely typification, institutionalization, and legitimation. That is, we human beings organize our observations about the world into categories or types. We do this as a way of making sense of the world. We create these types along religious, ethnic, racial, or other demographic lines. We create categories of health and mental health conditions into which we classify people. We divide others and ourselves according to types of interests, activities, political beliefs, geographical locations, and on and on. Berger and Luckmann (1966) note that we then over time institutionalize those types and structure our social functioning around them. In other words, we take the types or categories we have constructed and grant them a privileged role in our discourse. This in turn leads to the legitimation of these institutions as having some sort of power or reality on their own. Over time (whether years, centuries, or even millennia), we lose the awareness of how these types and institutions are themselves products of our own socially constructed narratives.

Think for example of recent cultural debates around marriage. When you read that word—*marriage*—tune in to your associations to it. What do you think, feel, and imagine? Ask yourself what your sense is of the place or role of marriage in society. Consider the intense and often heated discourse that has unfolded in the United States and in other countries as well about the "definition of marriage" and who should have access to it legally, religiously, and otherwise. Marriage is an institution in cultures around the world. But this social and cultural institution is also a *type* in Berger and Luckmann's (1966) language, and our understanding(s) of marriage are socially constructed. The meaning and role of marriage and the way it is lived out vary in different social and cultural contexts. In these contexts, marriage as a *type* is institutionalized and thereby legitimized. In other words, marriage is what we say it is because that is the tradition that has been handed down to us, and that is what we believe. Hence, altering this kind of social construction is commonly a slow-moving, complex process.

By way of summing up, Freedman and Combs (1996) have suggested that this social constructionist perspective leads to four key ideas: "(1) Realities are socially constructed. (2) Realities are constructed through language. (3) Realities are organized and maintained through narrative. (4) There are no essential truths" (p. 22). That last assertion may be particularly striking to you. Are we really saying that there is nothing that is really "true" (Spence, 1982)? Nothing that is knowable? Not exactly.

The balance, I would suggest, comes in the humility with which we pursue understanding of any dimension of life and experience, and the lightness with which we hold onto our sense of truth—particularly when it comes to the way in which human beings make meaning out of their experience. For example, we might take a rather smug and dismissive view of our scientific ancestors who somehow convinced themselves that the world is flat. We might remind ourselves how much more we know and how much more we have observed about the universe, and in so doing tell ourselves that we now *know* the way things are. But the truth, if you will, is that we now know only what we now know. We need to be aware that, for all of our advances, we have no idea what yet remains to be discovered, or how our knowledge and understanding will evolve over centuries to come. Similarly, members of societies that think of themselves as relatively "advanced" might be tempted to adopt an attitude of superiority over other cultures they consider to be less developed.

One of the gifts that we have been given by the discipline of anthropology is to be able to experience and hopefully understand diverse cultures on their own terms, and to consider life and the world from their perspective. While we remain nonetheless free to disagree and to maintain our own system of beliefs, this kind of cross-cultural understanding can do a great deal to foster empathy, cooperation, and even social justice. From a social work point of view, that is of course exceedingly valuable.

On a more directly interpersonal level, when we come face to face with another human person, we cannot pretend that we know all there is to know about them, or that any one single theory tells us everything there is to be known. Even as we consider our own subjective life experience, we must humbly realize that our sense of our very selves is limited by time, history, culture, gender, socioeconomic status, sexual orientation, and more—and the deeply powerful mutual interaction of all of these. Furthermore, when we, as social workers, open ourselves to the life experience of another human being, we automatically bring the biases and limitations that are part and parcel of our own limited experience of life and the world. I suggest that we need not think of this as a flaw to be overcome, however, as much as an inevitable dimension of personhood and one of which we must be continually aware. In order to practice effectively, it is of great benefit if we are deeply curious about the mystery of the person before us.

Consider this example. When I work with students in social work practice class or in clinical supervision to learn the skills of active listening and empathy, students readily acknowledge that they must suspend judgment and avoid telling clients what to do. That's pretty clear, even when we're beginners. Yet, time and time again I've gotten them to engage in role-playing around these skills and then listened to how frustrated they became. "I told myself I wasn't going to give advice. I wasn't going to judge. I was just really going to listen. And yet there I was five minutes in, telling the client what to do!" That in and of itself, I suggest, is an important lesson. It is challenging to be in touch enough with our own story and perspective to suspend it, hold it in awareness as if off to the side, and really listen to the story of another. It is challenging to trust that if I am patient and attentive I will understand more as I listen more. This is not to say that we will never respond or intervene. But as I hope you will discover throughout this book, narrative theory and practice suggest that my interventions will be deeper and more helpful if I listen attentively to the story of the client.

For this reason, one of the things that I hope comes through most clearly and powerfully throughout this book is the delicacy that is required of us as clinical social workers as we sit with, listen to, and interact with the complexity of the human stories that we are privileged to hear in our work. Each encounter we have with a client is a meeting of worlds—those of the client and the social worker. As a social worker, you are the instrument of your work. If you have been in practice for some time you know this to be true. At times you will work with clients who might appear quite different from you. At other times, they will seem quite similar. They may be people we wish to befriend, or people we don't honestly like. We may struggle to understand them or feel an instantaneous connection.

With each and every client, the discipline of our profession calls us to be self-aware and to notice what is evoked in us as we attend to the client. To help us in this regard, we may rely on both the classic and the developing scholarly literature on countertransference and the role it plays in the therapeutic relationship (Counselman, 2014; Lia, 2017; Oelsner, 2013; Viderman, 2010; Wolstein, 1988). We pay attention to the ways that our own story, particularly our own biases, may be evoked, and we do our utmost to contain them so that they interfere less with our ability to be open to the unfolding story of the person in front of us. We also seek to develop our awareness of what the very act of coming together with another person for help means in our cultural narratives. All of this remains true whether we work with individuals, families, groups, communities, or organizations.

Let's consider another example. A social worker at a local mental health clinic is scheduled to conduct an intake with a 52-year-old woman named Jessica who states that she would like to talk about some struggles she has been having. When they meet, the client tells the social worker that she has been feeling depressed for some time. For more than a month, she has been feeling pervasively sad, helpless, and hopeless. She has little energy and, though she has continued to function in a basic way, feels that she has been lacking motivation. The client notes that while she has been feeling quite bad over these past weeks, she has struggled with depression throughout most of her adult life. Most of the time she is able to keep the sadness at bay, but sometimes it feels overwhelming—like now.

As the social worker listens more deeply, she hears the client talk about her view of life and the world. Life is all about struggle, she thinks. No matter what you do you can never really get ahead. No matter how hard you try, it will all end up being pointless. The client notes that though she has some casual friendships, there is no one really close to her. She was married for 6 years in her 30s, but that ended in a contentious divorce. She has two children who are mostly wrapped up in their own lives. Fundamentally, she believes that the reason things never work out for her is that she does not deserve happiness. There must be something wrong with her as a person since she has had more than her fair share of hardship.

At this point, I'd like to invite you to pause and tune in to what you are thinking and feeling about this client. What else do you imagine about her? Do you have a mental picture of her? Some fantasy about the underlying causes of her painful depression? What else do you need to know about her, her history, and her social world to have a fuller understanding of what she is going through? And what difference would that information make?

For example, imagine how you might respond to her story if she had been raised in foster care on the one hand, or in a comfortable home with a large family on the other. Imagine if she were socioeconomically disadvantaged or financially well off. Imagine if she were Caucasian, or African-American, or Latina, or Asian. What if she identified as heterosexual, or lesbian, or transgender? What if she had experienced trauma or oppression and discrimination?

All human experience emerges from a multifaceted context that takes into account not only the characteristics with which we are born into the world, but also the ways in which the social environment conditions and shapes our development.

And in order to make meaning of all that experience, human beings continually tell stories—stories of *our self, the world, and our self in the world*. This is a phrase that I often use and that I find to be helpful in understanding narrative in sociocultural context. It captures for me the dynamic interplay between the individual and the environment in a way that is deeply important if we are to tap into the multilayered construction and meaning of our clients' stories.

A number of theorists have discussed this human disposition to tell stories as a means of understanding experience and relating it to others. Sarbin (1986), for example, refers to the storied nature of human conduct. That is, while our direct experience of the world may not, in and of itself, unfold as a story, any attempt we make to relate that experience to others or even reflect on it compels us to frame that experience along the lines of a story. We give it a beginning, a middle, and an ending, even if only an imagined one. This structure undergirds our efforts to make meaning of the mass of perceptions that first constitutes and that we continually integrate into our story of self, life, and the world (Polkinghorne, 1988).

Crossley (2000, 2003) has also elaborated upon the way in which we make meaning out of events by organizing them into an ordered sequence. This, she suggests, occurs along two lines. The first is temporal—the laying out of events chronologically. The second is relational. We look for the connections between events and try to understand the ways in which different pieces of our experience relate to each other and fit into the overall schema of our life. Crossley (2003) notes that language, in both its psychological and sociological dimensions, is the key building block of this effort. For this reason, one of the elements that lie at the core of a narrative approach to practice is a keen attention to the language clients use as they relate their story as well as the way in which the movement of the story unfolds. Saari (1991) comments,

> A story contains a structure and an order of meaning that the events of the real world do not possess even if they are considered in temporal sequence. A pure chronology lists in order of sequence every event that may have occurred in a particular arena regardless of its importance or relevance to anything. In contrast, a story selects temporally ordered events according to their causal relevance for a particular end point. (p. 139)

In keeping with the social constructionist foundations of narrative it is essential to remember that human stories always unfold in the context of the social and cultural worlds in which we live (Neimeyer, 2005). None of us recounts our experience in a vacuum. When we think of and connect emotionally to our story, and when we relate that story to the world, we do so in ways that we hope will be received, understood, and embraced by the world around us. When this does not happen we may feel isolated and misunderstood. Most, if not all, of us have had some experience with feeling misunderstood in this way. However, there are many for whom the pain that results when their narrative is not endorsed by the culture is an enormous burden reflected in the experience of marginalization and oppression.

If I suffer from what we more or less consensually refer to in the industrialized world as a "mental illness," I may have any one of a number of ways of understanding what that means (McTighe, 2015). I may think of it as a biological illness. I may think I am "crazy." I may view myself as under a curse or spell of some sort. I may also think that I have been misunderstood and labeled in a way that marginalizes and oppresses me. I may believe any of these things because others around me or in the world at large have communicated them to me. These varied interpretations will have a great deal to do with social and cultural factors like age, education, socioeconomic status, race and ethnicity, gender, and sexual orientation. They are also open to reconfiguration over time and with exposure to new information. This is one of the reasons we believe that a key intervention in the treatment of mental illness is psychoeducation.

It must be noted, however, that this capacity for an evolution of understanding (or narrative) applies not only to individuals and families, but also to culture itself. Even in the Western world, think of how our understanding of mental health and illness has evolved over centuries. So too has our response to it. We have moved from a time of possession and exorcisms to exile and institutionalization in asylums, to assertive community treatment. Even our language has evolved. Consider that pejorative words like *lunatic* were once used as clinical terms when our best understanding suggested that mental illness was somehow connected to the phases of the moon. Similarly, I have noted elsewhere (McTighe, 2015) that the antiquated diagnostic label of *hysteria* comes from the Greek word for uterus—*huster*. This was rooted in the cultural understanding of the nineteenth century that the etiology of the symptoms of *hysteria* was connected to female anatomy and hormonal cycles. On a social and cultural level, it came to serve as a means (intended or unintended) of marginalizing and minimizing women and their emotional experience.

Jerome Bruner (1986, 1987, 1990, 1991) is among the scholars who have made the greatest contribution to our understanding of this relationship between narrative and culture. He comments that there is a reflexive relationship between narrative and culture such that culture shapes our narratives, and narratives in turn shape the culture (Bruner, 1991). In other words, the narrative that each of us constructs as individuals is shaped by the social and cultural context in which we live. We then as individuals have a hand, however small, in shaping the culture that surrounds us.

If you want to know this is true, think about conversation among adolescents. This is a key place where language evolves and new expressions are born. These expressions are not only tied to age, however. They depend on racial, ethnic, and socioeconomic factors as well. They vary from inner cities to suburbs, and even regionally around the country and world. If you are not part of that cultural context, the interaction between young people may actually be quite hard to understand. Commonly though, these forms of expression start making their way through the broader culture around them. This is partly because adolescents bring their speech with them as they age, but also because they have an impact on families, groups, and the wider society. As these new forms of speech make their way through the culture, they often actually lose their appeal to the group from which they sprang.

When I try to make this point to my students in class, I will sometimes start talking without explanation in some form of really outdated slang. Since there is usually a great deal of diversity among my students I may use expressions that are not common in my culture of origin. Almost inevitably the students will start to laugh. I tell them to pause and ask themselves why they're laughing. They will start off by saying things like "No one says that anymore!" They will usually then comment that they didn't expect someone "like me" (i.e., of my age, race, ethnicity, education, and so forth …) to talk that way. What they tune into pretty quickly is an insight that is so deeply ingrained in us that we don't even think about it—language and narrative belong to culture—culture that shapes us and that we in turn shape by the way we live and embody it. When they perceive me as outside the culture reflected by that speech act, they do not expect me to express myself in that way.

Bruner (1991) takes his comments on this phenomenon even further by noting that culture itself provides us with a shared set of meanings—like a narrative menu. On the one hand, this offers us a range of options for narrative self-expression. On the other hand, it limits in some sense our choices, not only for how we relate or communicate our experience, but also of how we understand that experience in the first place. Of course a culture is made up of any number of subcultures and can allow for a multiplicity of possible meanings. All one needs to do is watch a political debate during an election year to witness the way in which groups of people from a broadly similar culture espouse divergent interpretations of the same events. If we consider this on a more granular level, we may note that not only different political parties have different narratives of the political scene, but so too do different regions, socioeconomic groups, genders, ethnic and racial groups, etc. We saw this dynamic at work clearly in the 2016 US Presidential election. Political polling can become extraordinarily complex as each campaign tries to understand how their narrative or message is playing with all of the cultural subgroups.

Anthropologists work at decoding and cataloging the ways in which diverse cultures make sense of experience. They may spend years listening and observing in order to capture the nuance of words, gestures, rituals, and other forms of cultural expression. I suggest that a good deal of the fascination in this is the seemingly infinite number of way human beings have of making sense of and constructing their worlds. And from this, whether in a faraway land or much closer to home, the narratives of human life and experience flow.

In line with this thinking, Howard (1991) has suggested that culture is itself the consensus developed in community about how to make meaning of experience. The implications of this for the practice of social work are significant. Saleeby (1994) notes that in our work we stand at the intersection of the meaning-making systems of the client, the worker, and the culture at large. This is true whether we work with individuals, families, groups, organizations, or communities. On each of these levels, he suggests, part of our responsibility as social workers is to tune into the ways narratives may emerge from and even support oppressive structures in the social environment, and to challenge these for the betterment of our clients. From a narrative research perspective, Josselson (1995) notes that narratives are records of the meaning-making systems of human persons and that attending to narrative is a means to understanding how people make sense of the world.

When discussing the social constructionist foundations of narrative earlier, I acknowledged that these might raise in the minds of some the question of whether there is anything knowable or true. This applies not only to the overarching scheme of life and the world as a whole, but also to the individual person who is struggling to make sense of their experience and understand their own identity in context. Bruner (1987) offers a powerful insight about this.

> The heart of my argument is this: eventually the culturally shaped cognitive and linguistic processes that guide the self-telling of life narratives achieve the power to structure perceptual experience, to organize memory, to segment and purpose-build the very "events" of life. In the end, we *become* the autobiographical narratives by which we "tell about" our lives. (p. 15)

This is the dynamic we see in clients, families, and even communities when the story they tell of themselves, the world, and themselves in the world has become so embedded in their very sense of self that even entertaining an alternative seems like an impossibility.

A similar distinction has been referred to as the difference between grand lives or narratives and "small stories"—the countless everyday narratives in all their own complexity that make up what we think of as our "real life" (Bamberg, 2004; Georgakopolou, 2006). From a research point of view, and I would argue from a clinical one as well, attending to the small stories that people tell over time offers access to a deeper and we might say more authentic version of the narrative of their identity (Bamberg, 2004). We look not just for one story or interpretation of an event, but for the patterns of how meaning is constructed from their experience.

Spence (1982) has offered a now classic treatment of what is meant by "truth" in the psychoanalytic situation. Whether or not one is psychoanalytically oriented in their thinking, his insights remain important. Spence makes a distinction between historical truth (the way in which we typically think of what is true—a sequential unfolding of events as they "really" happened) and the narrative weaving of events that takes place in the clinical context as a social worker listens to the story of the client. There is of course an inevitable subjective quality to these narratives, and our hope as clinicians is that they will evolve over time (Schafer, 1980, 1992). And they do. However, this question of what is true can be a stumbling block for us as clinicians as we try to make sense of what we are hearing from our clients. We may find ourselves listening to clients and asking ourselves, "Did that *really* happen? Did it happen *that way*?" We may hear client's stories and have a different sense of their meaning than the client does. We may feel, or even know, at times that we are being *lied* to. The challenge for us clinically, I would suggest, is not to get into a tug-of-war over what is true. Rather, we listen to and receive the client's story as *their* story, and wonder with them about what it means and how this came to be so. These may be stories of great pain or unrealistic triumph. They may tell us of the unfairness of the world or of having been mistreated by those around them. Sometimes, as clinicians, we may feel that the client is trying to manipulate us into responding a certain way based on the narrative that they share.

When I was a social work student I had a wonderful supervisor who was perhaps one of the most grounded social workers I have ever met. Her name is Linda. By all accounts (and by my observation on a couple of occasions), Linda was extraordinarily skilled at working with clients diagnosed with Borderline Personality Disorder (itself a narrative, cultural construction—though one that has explanatory power for a dimension of human suffering). Clients diagnosed as borderline are notorious for challenging boundaries and trying to manipulate those around them—including their therapists. Many clinicians speak of them as difficult to work with and to be avoided if possible (also a narrative). I once asked Linda what she thought made her so successful with these clients whom so many viewed as simply impossible. With a good dose of humility I'm sure, Linda said that she always tried to see beyond all of those off-putting interpersonal qualities and ask herself, "What is it that has happened to this person that has made them feel that this is what they need to do in the world to have their needs met?" In this way, she didn't need to feel compelled to retaliate or to violate her own boundaries or her sense of what her work was about. But she could also understand with empathy the effort the client was making to be taken care of in the best way he or she knew how.

Though Linda did not frame this understanding along the lines of narrative, I am suggesting that one way of understanding Linda's profound insight is to see the client's challenging behavior as the expression of a narrative about a world that has been erratic and painfully disappointing. Now many years later, one of the things I often tell students and supervisees I work with is, "It's hard to be manipulated if you know you might be being manipulated." That may sound odd at first, but think about it for a moment. One of the reasons that clinicians often become frustrated and angry with clients is that they are engaged with the client in the kind of "tug-of-war" I referred to earlier. In their effort to get at "the truth," and their concern that they are being lied to, they are having a hard time listening to the unfolding narrative of the client.

Alternatively, they have adopted the client's point of view as "the truth" in some immutable sense, and then feel resentful or betrayed if things do not turn out to be just as they had been portrayed. This is the time for listening with suspended judgment—for hearing the client's experience *as* their experience and for trying to engage the client in wondering about it and transforming it together. As Josselson (1995) notes, "Narratives are not records of facts, of how things were, but of a meaning-making system that makes sense out of the chaotic mass of perceptions and experiences of a life" (p.33). In other words, the client tells the story they have constructed. Together the client and the social worker must tell the story they co-construct through the treatment (Neimeyer, 1993; Saari, 1991).

This brings us to the work of Michael White (1948–2008). White was an Australian social worker whose work has become almost synonymous with what most people think of as narrative therapy, particularly in the world of family therapy. Though the field of narrative is, as you probably now can sense, much broader and more diverse than the work of any one individual or even discipline, White's work did an enormous amount to put narrative on the map and to help us attend to the impact of story on our sense of life and experience.

Together with his colleague David Epston, White (1990) agreed with the notion that we structure our experience along the lines of a story. He made explicit though that we do this in a selective way. White and Epston offer the concept of dominant story lines to emphasize the way in which human beings attend selectively to certain aspects of their experience while subjugating or minimizing others. These dominant story lines work their way into our speech when we hear generalizing statements that begin with phrases like "I'm the kind of person who …; I never …; I always …; The world is …; People are …; Life is …." This is akin to Bruner's (1987) perspective on the ways in which autobiographical narratives can constrain our sense of self.

For example, let's come back to the client, Jessica, whom I described earlier. I noted that Jessica believes that life is all about struggle, and that no matter what she does or how hard she tries, she will never be able to get ahead. After all, there is something fundamentally wrong with her as a person. White and Epston (1990) would suggest that this talk is reflective of Jessica's dominant story line. Undoubtedly, many frustrating and disappointing experiences have together given rise to this story of the difficulty of life and the futility of effort. This problem-saturated story, as White and Epston would call it, limits Jessica's view of herself as well as what is possible. Without intending to do so, other aspects of life that do not conform to the dominant story line are dismissed as irrelevant or not even noticed. Note how very much in line this is with Bruner's thinking. Her narrative about herself and her life has limited the very parameters within which she can experience life.

Let's imagine for example that alongside the painful and frustrating experiences that reinforce Jessica's dominant story line, other things are also happening. Perhaps Jessica has a strong circle of long-time friends who care deeply about her. Maybe Jessica is highly skilled at her work, and has done well in her company, gaining not only financial compensation but sincere praise as well. And perhaps the way in which her children are wrapped up in their own lives is reflective of what we might view as their developmentally appropriate phase of life, and not so much an uncaring dismissal of their mother. What any seasoned clinician knows is that even if there is significant evidence for all of these more positive statements, it may nonetheless be extremely difficult for Jessica to hear and embrace them.

This is where we must come back to the importance of not engaging in a tug-of-war with the client. In our sincere effort to help Jessica "feel better" we might be tempted to suggest that she, in one way or another, simply look on the bright side! Since we can see so many things that are "positive," we may wrestle with her over what is in fact "true." In our desire to be encouraging, we risk communicating a real lack of empathy for Jessica. We might even start to label her as defensive and help rejecting. And for her part, Jessica may be left feeling that we just don't get it.

In this situation, White and Epston (1990) might suggest that what is needed is a process of deconstruction and reconstruction. This entails listening to the story, externalizing the problem, and deconstructing the dominant story line. It is quite common for clients not to have any real conscious awareness of the presence of this story line or its impact on their life and sense of self. Helping the client to see and hear it as a narrative can itself be a powerful intervention.

From there White and Epston suggest exploring for and reintroducing what they refer to as "subjugated truths"—those aspects of experience that are *also true*. Note that by highlighting them as also true, we are not battling with the client over the truth of their own perceptions. Rather, they advocate listening carefully and working patiently with clients to shift that dominant story line gradually to incorporate aspects of their experience that are more life giving. This is, of course, only a thumbnail sketch of White's perspective. He has developed a number of tools and strategies for implementing these insights in clinical work with individuals and families (White, 2007).

Another word about the notion of "*also true*." In my clinical experience, some clients at first may hear this as superficially selecting a different version of reality if your view of the current one doesn't suit you. In other words, if you don't like the way things are, just tell yourself they are different. This of course lacks depth and will not be helpful. It is also not at all the point of narrative. In narrative work, we are not inviting the client simply to "think about it differently." Rather, we sensitively and compassionately listen to as much of the fullness of their experience as we can reach, and together with them contemplate how that story has been socially constructed and what parts of it are being subjugated. We then wonder about what else is legitimately true. This neither compels the client to live in some sort of fantasyland, nor tells them that their understanding of their experience is wrong. Our goal is to help clients integrate *more* of the truth of their experience and to do so in a way that is healing and life giving.

Because I see this kind of narrative process as organic and one that unfolds in a unique way for each client, I do not believe that there is any cookie cutter approach to narrative practice that is ultimately helpful. However, I have over the years discovered general ways of helping clients become more attuned to their narratives and the ways in which these impact their life.

The first of these has to do with the fundamental stance of the social worker toward the client and their story. Earlier I suggested that to practice effectively, we must be deeply curious about the mystery of the person before us. As every practicing clinician knows, if I have sat with hundreds of people whom we might broadly describe as "depressed," and even if I can discern commonalities and patterns in their presentation that I take to be diagnostic, every one of those individuals has been unique and their story has been distinctive. I advocate then adopting an attitude of wonderment as we approach each person, a stance that opens me up to discovering who they understand themselves to be. In supervision, as supervisees try to make sense of all of their impressions of a client, I often remind them to take it all in as information. What you hear (and don't), what you see, how you feel when you're with the client (whatever that is), how you experience them engaging with you (or not), and fantasies and associations that the client's story conjure in you all offer rich information about the client and the story that is beginning to unfold between you. Be curious. Wonder about them and about what you are experiencing in their presence.

It is of course true that as social workers we are subject to the constraints of time as well as all the demands of our professional ethics. We are responsible for thoughtful, accurate assessment. We strive to make helpful interventions that will assist the client in achieving his or her goals. Narrative asks us not to put aside these responsibilities, but to trust that a deep posture of listening to the client's story will help us do just that. If we allow the client to transport us, metaphorically speaking, into the heart of their story, we will understand more and may be even more effective. We will then be able to enter into the story with them in the space of our treatment and help them discover even more as the narrative unfolds.

At times, it may be important to help stimulate "storytelling" on the part of the client. Just as we may help socialize a client to any form of treatment, we can also encourage them to engage with us on a narrative basis (though we may never refer explicitly to this as an approach). Our curiosity, our questions, and our responses can encourage clients to be attentive both to the story they have crafted thus far and to the story that is continually unfolding and in which we will be privileged to have a role as their therapist.

Particularly when I am trying to assist a client in going deeper or envisioning something different about their story, I will encourage them to "play" with me a bit (Winnicott, 1971) as we wonder about the narrative together. "And then what would happen?" or "How would you like the story to unfold?" I may suggest that we externalize the narrative and imagine the story and its arc as we would a film or novel. "What do you think might happen then? What else might the character be thinking or feeling?"

We may find that clients respond with what I call the "reflexive 'I don't know.'" This happens when, in response to some inquiry on our part, a client responds immediately, almost automatically, "I don't know." I have known many a therapist who simply moves on, taking that response as a dead end. I would encourage a bit more persistence. It is of course possible that a client doesn't really know. But we can attempt to move gently past whatever automatic block may be represented by that "I don't know." We might encourage the client to sit with it for a moment and tune in to what is going on inside.

At other times I may encourage clients to draw from their own unconscious resources by simply "making it up" in order to help stimulate their thinking. This serves as a starting point for reflection, not an end point. It is important to remember what I noted earlier. This is not about simply selecting a more pleasant fantasy and trying to convince ourselves that it is real. It is, rather, reminiscent of Bollas' (1987) notion of the unthought known, that aspect of experience that we *do* know on some deep level but that we have not thematized for ourselves and about which we have not yet been able to think. As clients learn to play with us in therapy, we can help them uncover aspects of their narrative that have been banished from awareness, or of which they were never consciously aware in the first place. In either case, it can greatly help our clients add depth and dimension to their narrative in a way that is life giving.

In light of all of this, and as we move forward with the rest of our considerations in this book, there are a few things I want to encourage you to keep in mind. Think of these summary points as tools for the journey:

1. All human experience is crafted along the lines of a story.
2. In addition to our biological inheritance, our stories are socially constructed and are shaped by perhaps countless variables such as history, geography, gender, race, ethnicity, language, socioeconomics, and education.
3. Narrative theory and practice serve as an extraordinarily powerful interpretive tool to help us, together with our clients, understand their experience more deeply.
4. Because our stories are bound up in culture and language, narrative theory and practice can unlock for our clients the potential, as we journey with them, to discover deeper and hidden dimensions to their narratives that may help them live with greater satisfaction and vitality.

5. For us as social workers, especially as we work with individuals, families, and groups that have been marginalized and oppressed, the power of narrative to help uncover new dimensions of experience can be a potent force for change in the lives of clients as well as society as a whole.

In each of the following chapters, we will look at a particular clinical issue or an aspect of human suffering and struggle that we commonly encounter as social workers. We will reflect on how we engage clients and their experience from a stance of empathy, healing, and social justice. We will also take into account what this all means for us personally and professionally. I encourage you to be thoughtful about the content of the theory and research that we will review together. I invite you to consider how they apply to the examples I will use throughout. Through them, I hope to make a narrative style of thinking and practicing come to life in a way that will help you in the work you do with your own clients and communities.

Questions and Activities for Discussion and Further Reflection

1. What do you see as the social and cultural factors that have the greatest negative impact on the clients with whom you work? How do you understand them as socially constructed?
2. What are the implications of a social constructionist point of view for a biopsychosociospiritual view of the human condition?
3. Identify a client with whom you are working and think about how you have conceptualized your client up to now. Try to reflect on your client and your work together from a narrative perspective. See if you can discern the narrative structure that runs through their story.
    (a) What do you see as the key elements of the story?
    (b) What are the social and cultural factors that have gone into shaping that story? How have they done so?
    (c) Does the narrative perspective help you see or understand anything new about your client and how you might approach your work with them?
4. Reflect on the narrative of your own life experience. Consider journaling about the people and experiences that have had a hand in the way your story has developed. What would you identify as your dominant story line(s)? Can you identify any aspects of your narrative that have evolved or shifted over time? What factors have led to that shift?
5. Do a role-play in class. Allow one student to take on the persona of the client. Another student can act as the social worker listening for the client's narrative as it unfolds. As a class, identify the social and cultural factors that have shaped their narrative, with particular emphasis on those that have resulted in marginalization and/or oppression.

References

Bamberg, M. (2004). Talk, small stories, and adolescent identities. *Human Development, 47*, 366–369.
Berger, P., & Luckmann, T. (1966). *The social construction of reality*. New York: Doubelday.
Bollas, C. (1987). *The shadow of the object: Psychoanalyis of the unthought known*. New York: Columbia University Press.
Bruner, J. (1986). *Actual minds, possible worlds*. Cambridge, MA: Harvard University Press.
Bruner, J. (1987). Life as narrative. *Social Research, 54*, 11–32.
Bruner, J. (1990). *Acts of meaning*. Cambridge, MA: Harvard University Press.
Bruner, J. (1991). The narrative construction of reality. *Critical Inquiry, 18*(1), 1–21.
Counselman, E. F. (2014). Containing and using powerful therapist reactions. In L. Motherwell & J. J. Shay (Eds.), *Complex dilemmas in group therapy: Pathways to resolution* (2nd ed., pp. 109–119). New York, NY: Routledge/Taylor & Francis Group.
Crossley, M. L. (2000). Narrative psychology, trauma and the study of self/identity. *Theory & Psychology, 10*(4), 527–546.
Crossley, M. L. (2003). Formulating narrative psychology: The limitations of contemporary social constructionism. *Narrative Inquiry, 13*(2), 287–300.
Freedman, J., & Combs, G. (1996). *Narrative therapy: The social construction of preferred realities*. New York: W.W. Norton.
Georgakopolou, A. (2006). Thinking big with small stories in narrative and identity analysis. *Narrative Inquiry, 16*(1), 122–130.
Gergen, K. J. (2015). *An invitation to social construction* (3rd ed.). Thousand Oaks, CA: Sage.
Howard, G. S. (1991). Culture tales: A narrative approach to thinking, cross-cultural psychology, and psychotherapy. *American Psychologist, 46*(3), 187–197.
Hyvarinen, M. (2010). Revisiting the narrative turns. *Life Writing, 7*(1), 69–82.
Josselson, R. (1995). Imagining the real: Empathy, narrative and the dialogic self. In R. Josselson & A. Lieblich (Eds.), *Interpreting experience: The narrative study of lives*. Thousand Oaks, CA: Sage.
Lia, M. (2017). Reflections, and relative examples, regarding countertransference, empathy, and observation. *International Forum of Psychoanalysis, 26*(2), 85–96. https://doi.org/10.1080/0803706X.2016.1200197
McTighe, J. P. (2015). Narratives of illness, difference, and personhood. In B. Probst (Ed.), *Critical thinking in clinical assessment and diagnosis* (pp. 171–188). New York: Springer.
Neimeyer, R. A. (1993). An appraisal of constructivist psychotherapies. *Journal of Consulting and Clinical Psychology, 61*(2), 221–234.
Neimeyer, R. A. (2005). Tragedy and transformation: Meaning reconstruction in the wake of traumatic loss. In S. Heilman (Ed.), *Death, bereavement, and mourning*. New Brunswick, NJ: Transaction Publishers.
Oelsner, R. (2013). *Transference and countertransference today*. New York, NY: Routledge/Taylor & Francis Group.
Polkinghorne, D. E. (1988). *Narrative knowing and the human sciences*. Albany, NY: State University of New York Press.
Riessman, C. K., & Quinney, L. (2005). Narrative in social work: A critical review. *Qualitative Social Work, 4*(4), 391–412.
Saari, C. (1991). *The creation of meaning in clinical social work*. New York: The Guilford Press.
Saleeby, D. (1994). Culture, theory, and narrative: The intersection of meanings in practice. *Social Work, 39*(4), 351–359.
Sarbin, T. R. (Ed.). (1986). *Narrative psychology: The storied nature of human conduct*. New York: Praeger.
Schafer, R. (1980). Narration in the psychoanalytic dialogue. *Critical Inquiry, 7*(1), 29–53.
Schafer, R. (1992). *Retelling a life: Narrative and dialogue in psychoanalysis*. New York: Basic Books.
Spence, D. P. (1982). *Narrative truth and historical truth*. New York: W.W. Norton.

References

Viderman, S. (2010). The role of the countertransference (1982). In D. Birksted-Breen, S. Flanders, & A. Gibeault (Eds.), *Reading French psychoanalysis* (pp. 210–217). New York, NY: Routledge/Taylor & Francis Group.

White, M. (2007). *Maps of narrative practice*. New York: W.W. Norton.

White, M., & Epston, D. (1990). *Narrative means to therapeutic ends*. New York: W.W. Norton.

Winnicott, D. W. (1971). *Playing and reality*. London: Tavistock Publications Ltd..

Wolstein, B. (1988). *Essential papers on countertransference*. New York, NY: New York University Press.

Chapter 2
Encountering the Self, Encountering the Other: Narratives of Race and Ethnicity

Guiding Questions

What does narrative theory have to tell us about race and ethnicity and its implications for clinical practice?
What do we mean by the term *Otherness* and how can narrative help us understand and engage it as social workers?
In what ways do race and ethnicity inform the developing sense of self of the individual in the social environment?
How may narrative help us to attend to the dynamics of race and ethnicity in the clinical encounter with our clients?

Think about the last time you filled out a form that asked for your demographic information. Perhaps it was at a doctor's office, at the department of motor vehicles, or on an application to a college or university. Maybe you were participating in the US Census. Depending on how old you are, you may have filled out these kinds of forms countless times. Now think specifically about a question that is on virtually every one of those forms—the one that asks about your race and ethnicity. Do you answer that question? It is usually not required and comes with a "prefer not to answer" option. If you don't answer, ask yourself why? What is your feeling about providing that sort of information? Do you find it irrelevant? Do you wonder what use the person, or in some cases the government, has for it? If you do answer, what is your answer? Is it an easy question for you to respond to? Does the form offer you a choice that corresponds to your sense of your identity? Have you resigned yourself to selecting the one that matches you most closely? Do you have any feelings about checking that little box? Were you able to select more than one if you needed to? Or were you forced to pick only one? Is the sense of identity behind your selection something that you have spent any significant amount of time considering? What has made that so? I am willing to wager that this may be the most time you have ever spent thinking about a question on a demographic form. What we are really tapping into, however, is something much more profound than a simple question on a form. It is a piece of the story of our self—of who we are.

Among the most fundamental dimensions of our identity as human persons are our race and ethnicity (Sue & Sue, 2016). And yet these ubiquitous categories, whether they appear on a census form, a college application, in a political debate, our public and private conversations, or in the immediate and inevitable judgments and appraisals we make of each other in our comings and goings, are themselves social constructions. Think about that. Race and ethnicity are social constructions. They are based on phenotypic differences in human genetics and human appearance, but it is we who have given them labels—labels that we imbue with deep and often divisive social meaning (Gomez, 2012). Though the DNA of all races and ethnicities is virtually identical, we invest them with a great deal of meaning in the social world.

The history of this is long and deep and its implications are extraordinarily far reaching, affecting us as a human community socially, politically, economically, geographically, and even romantically. It affects where we live, with whom we work, with whom we associate, and many times with whom we feel safe. For us in the United States, there is perhaps no greater wound that impacts our history and our present than racism. From the mindset that predated and lay the groundwork for slavery, through an era of lynchings and state-sanctioned segregation, to the violence and contrasting peaceful protests of the civil rights era, to the social and political unrest of today as we deal with conflict between police and communities and the debate over which lives matter, racism affects our culture in both overt and covert ways.

Of course, this reality is not unique to Americans. Racial and ethnic violence is found throughout the world in everything from personal attitudes to socially structured caste systems, to campaigns of ethnic cleansing. In many places in the world, socially constructed differences between ethnic communities that share the same geography have led to generations and sometimes centuries of animosity and strife (Baum, 2010; Nuttman-Shwartz, 2008). In this chapter, we take up the topic of narratives of race and ethnicity and try to understand both the dynamics of those narratives, our relationship to them individually and collectively, and in a more specific way their inevitable presence in and impact on the clinical social work situation. In the last chapter, we discussed the recursive relationship between our individual narratives and culture. That relationship shapes our experience of race and ethnicity in inescapable ways. For us as social workers, it is a profoundly important aspect of our personal and professional narrative—one that impacts our work whether with communities, organizations, groups, families, or individuals.

Let's begin by considering further the notion that race and ethnicity are social constructions. A number of authors have explored this idea and its implications for our history and social environment. We might first consider what we mean by race and ethnicity. Smedley and Smedley (2005) have noted that race has an ideological history that goes back at least until the late seventeenth century. This involved the establishment of a social and cultural hierarchy that related to the perceived worth of people of different races. In spite of the eventual scientific awareness of the absence of any biological or genetic distinction between races, what predominated in discourse and attitudes was the culturally invented sense of difference based on physical appearance and behavior. This view of difference was not a neutral observation, however. It brought with it beliefs about the inequality and separateness of races and consequent legal structures that facilitated everything from slavery to segregation.

As for the related construct of ethnicity, consider the following definition.

> Ethnicity refers to clusters of people who have common culture traits that they distinguish from those of other people. People who share a common language, geographic locale or place of origin, religion, sense of history, traditions, values, beliefs, food habits, and so forth, are perceived, and view themselves as constituting, an ethnic group. (Smedley & Smedley, 2005, p. 17)

Notice how this definition emphasizes human qualities that both draw people together into a community and set them apart from one another. This is the nature of our relationship to race and ethnicity. It informs in part our sense of our own identity as well as the category or categories into which we believe we do or do not fit in the social world.

So strong is this predilection to fit people into more or less neat categories, people developed what is referred to as the "one drop rule" (Rockquemore & Laszloffy, 2003; Smedley & Smedley, 2005). Emerging from the nineteenth century and encoded in law in the twentieth century, the one drop rule stated that if a person had even one black ancestor, they were considered black. The same applied to Native Americans. Not only did this rule reflect an intolerance of racial diversity, it also assigned to such individuals an inferior social standing with all of the consequences that came along with it. It is important for us to note the socially constructed nature of this kind of categorization. We are surrounded by this notion of race with all of its political and social ramifications (Lawrence, 2012), and we find therein the roots of our narrative of race and ethnicity.

For individuals who identify as multiracial or biracial, the meaning of race may be experienced as even more complex, since in the co-constructed and reflexive relationship between individual and communal narratives they may find themselves struggling to discern a sense of racial identity that they experience as authentic (Keddell, 2009) and that they may not find mirrored in the world around them (Rockquemore & Laszloffy, 2003). From a narrative point of view, such individuals may find themselves in a process of "rejecting constraining narratives and identifying with empowering narratives" as they develop a sense of their own identity that is "constructive, functional, and affirming of their experiences" (Hill & Thomas, 2000, p. 196).

Narrative is a powerful tool and approach to understand issues of race, ethnicity, and the development of identity. Consider that, for example, throughout our history belonging to a racial or ethnic minority has brought with it the experience of marginalization, and an identity that has been pathologized, with the only remedy being as complete an integration as possible into mainstream culture (Stonequest, 1935). In response to this, a concept of ethnic identity development emerged that was based on a stage model. This model typically saw members from racial and ethnic minority groups as beginning with an initial stance of unquestioned or negative identity or sense of self. As they developed, these individuals would move through a period of self-exploration and critique of the dominant Euro-American perspective toward a progressively greater degree of acceptance of their racial and ethnic identity (Yi & Shorter-Gooden, 1999).

In contrast to this, a narrative perspective views the development of racial and ethnic identity as taking place in relational context and unfolding in numerous and highly individualized ways for each person. Narrative encourages a view of identity as continually emerging in tandem with the unique body of experience of each individual in social context (Polkinghorne, 1988). This attention to the personal story and developing identity of each person is what allows all of us to challenge the master narratives of race and ethnicity that are handed down (if not to say imposed) upon us in favor of stories of racial and ethnic identity that are multivalent and more uniquely tailored to the self of the individual (Godley & Loretto, 2013).

This has implications for our social work practice and for our commitment to social justice since members of racial and ethnic minorities with whom we work are more likely to feel invisible, particularly in new and unfamiliar social contexts (Pyne & Means, 2013). As we attend to the nature and meaning of their own racial and ethnic identity, to where they are on that journey, and to the factors that have influenced that developmental process, we signal to our clients that we see them; we hear them; and we are open to them. But we do something else equally as profound. We dare to open ourselves to discovering more about who we are and to what may occur in the unique process that unfolds within and between us. Whether in the intimacy of the relationship between therapist and client, or the larger arena of advocacy with organizations and communities, this kind of openness, I suggest, lies at the heart of a genuine pursuit of justice.

In spite of this, in big and small ways, the challenge of openness for us as human beings has been a daunting one. A particular way of conceptualizing this that I often discuss with my students is the predilection we seem to have to identify and separate out the "other." As we have been discussing, the "other" may be anyone who doesn't look like me, sound like me, think like me, relate like me, agree with me, and on and on … (Aymer, 2016; Baum, 2011; Ploesser & Mecheril, 2012). This focus on otherness lies at the root of human divisions by focusing on difference and separateness, ignoring or perhaps fearing to seek out those things that may bring us together.

Let me offer an example to illustrate what I mean. Many years ago I had the opportunity to work for a year as an intern in the jail of a major city on the East Coast of the United States. The facility was massive, loud, and dank. The first time I walked in, passed through the metal detector, and approached the officer who would pat me down (a procedure that would be repeated every time I entered and left the jail) I was both exhilarated and terrified. A part of me wondered if I was in over my head. I had a wonderful supervisor named Mike who was dedicated, encouraging, and reassuring. I learned the ropes quickly enough and got started on my work with the residents, which would consist of brief counseling and support. The population of the jail was over 95% African-American. There were almost no Caucasians among the residents. Most were incarcerated for offenses involving drugs, theft, and violence, even murder.

I've found that many people aren't aware of the theoretical distinction between a jail and a prison; I certainly wasn't. It was one of the first things my supervisor taught me. Jail is meant to be a temporary facility where individuals are held following arrest while they await trial. If they are convicted of a crime, they will serve out their sentence in a prison. At the end of their sentence, they may also spend time in a jail as a step down while they await release. In other words, jails are meant to be temporary while prisons are meant for longer term incarceration.

I referred above to the *theoretical* distinction between jail and prison. That is because in point of fact, people are sometimes held in jails for years. Court systems are overburdened and can be painfully slow. Correctional facilities are overcrowded and beds are at a premium wherever they may be found. As you might imagine, any jail is a harsh place. But these factors lead to environments where the level noise is almost assaultive, and the tension and perceived danger in the air are palpable. Discipline is structured around following procedures and rules, and this can bring with it great deal of impersonalization, anonymity, and invisibility. Often enough, I felt as though the only contribution I was making in my work was to offer a few moments of nonthreatening attention to the human being who was before me.

Among my responsibilities at the jail was the task of visiting the locked ward of the hospital that was next door. This was where prisoners were taken who required in-patient hospital care. They were housed on a special unit that was behind locked doors with armed corrections officers guarding the entrance. As one entered the unit, there were a few private rooms followed by a large open area with approximately 20 beds. One Monday morning when I arrived I greeted a nurse who was on duty and asked if there was anything in particular I could do to be helpful. She asked if I would speak to the man in the first private room. He had been brought in on Saturday immediately following his arrest. They needed to be able to connect an I.V. for him, but he would not let anyone touch him. They had been working on it since Saturday and were frustrated. They didn't know what else to do shy of restraining him. I told her I would see what I could do.

I entered the room to find the curtains drawn and a small lamp lit next to the bed. A young black man lay there, curled in the fetal position, his back to me. He wore only a pair of gray shorts. I could see that he had bandages over his eyes and the front of his head. I knew only that his name was Ronald. I greeted him in a quiet tone and introduced myself. He did not respond, and yet somehow I was certain that he wasn't asleep. I tried asking him if there was anything he needed, but again there was no response. Not sure what to do, I contemplated leaving the room. I could tell Ronald that I'd be happy to come back if he changed his mind. He need only tell the nurse. But there was something else about the moment that told me not to go. He needed someone there, even though he seemed so far away.

Unsure how to make a connection with a man who could not see me even if he would look at me, I hesitantly asked if it would be ok if I put my hand on his arm. Though my way of practicing would never ordinarily involve physical contact with a client, apart from a possible hand shake that I usually wait for the client to initiate, I didn't know what else to do. To my surprise he nodded yes. I gently placed my hand on his forearm. He exhaled. After a moment in silence, I said to him,

> "Ronald, it seems to me like you're in so much pain. Can you tell me what happened to you?"
> "I got shot," he whispered.
> "You were shot?" I repeated, half out of shock and half to confirm that I had heard him correctly. "What happened?"

Ronald went on to tell me that he was an enforcer and collector for a local drug dealer. Somehow the drug dealer had become convinced that Ronald was stealing from him. Early in the morning on Saturday, as Ronald was sleeping alone in his apartment, another collector arrived with a gun to get the money back. Ronald said that he was awakened from sleep to the shouts of the other man, "Where's the money? Where's the money?" Ronald was confused and tried to get up, when the other man fired. He told me he was shot at point blank range in the face with a .357 magnum pistol. The bullets took both of Ronald's eyes. A piece of the front of his skull was shattered though the bullet didn't penetrate his brain. Another bullet grazed the side of his left nostril leaving a small hole. When he was brought to the hospital by ambulance, there was nothing doctors could do to save his eyes. A steel plate was placed in the front of his head and he was stitched up. He was swollen and bruised and in tremendous pain. And he was terrified.

I was speechless. My hand still on his forearm, I finally said, "Ronald. It's a miracle you're alive." Over the next 10 or 15 min, we talked about what he needed right then in the moment. He was unsure what was going on, and had been afraid each time someone came in the room. Of course, he could not see who it was. I explained that the nurses needed to connect him to an I.V. to give him the medicine the doctor had ordered. He reluctantly agreed, and asked if I would stay in the room while they did it. The nurse was surprised, of course, when I went to tell her that he had consented to the I.V.. Ronald held my hand as the nurse inserted the needle. He allowed her to put a pillow behind his head and he sat up in the bed. He said that he would eat for the first time in 2 days.

Before I left his room that morning, I assured Ronald that I would be back and that we would talk again. I gave him my schedule and let him know when he could expect me to visit. A couple of days later, I returned to work and was surprised to learn that Ronald had been discharged from the hospital and was being held in the infirmary of the jail. This was partly due to his medical condition, and partly for his safety. Ronald was blind now and was in no position to protect himself in the general population of the jail. I went to the infirmary and found him sitting in a typical orange jumpsuit on the edge of the cot in his cell. From the entrance of the cell I greeted him. He was happy I had come and invited me to sit. I sat down next to him on the cot and we spoke for some time.

I continued to visit him two or three times a week for the next several weeks. During those sessions I learned a great deal about him. He was raised in the city by a single mother. They were poor, sometimes hungry, surrounded by violence, drugs, and crime, and Ronald saw few options in his life. He became involved with drugs, which led to robbery—even from his own mother, breaking into her apartment and stealing electronics, and jewelry—anything he could sell on the street for drugs. Eventually, he went to work for the drug dealer. Sitting next to me on that cot, Ronald described in detail a life of drugs and guns, collections gone wrong, the aftermath of shootings he had witnessed and perpetrated, and the unraveling of his relationship to his boss, a man he feared was still pursuing him through the contacts he had in the jail population. As I went to bed at night, in the safety of my home just a few miles from that jail, I would think about Ronald's story, and mine.

Ronald and I were both 25 years old at that time. I am white. He is black. I was raised in an intact middle to lower middle class family in another city, in a neighborhood where there was little crime. As a boy growing up in the city, I certainly knew about crime and it had come close to my life, but it was something I mostly associated with *other* people—other neighborhoods, other communities, and yes, other races and ethnicities. A single mother (of whom he spoke highly) raised Ronald in poverty. She was a woman who did her best to provide—to counteract the harshness of the world around her and Ronald. But for whatever combination of reasons, it didn't save Ronald. I was a graduate student who was looking forward to a professional career and wondering what the future would hold for me. Ronald had dropped out of high school and knew even at that time that incarceration was likely in his future. It was now in his present.

So how did it happen that my narrative had unfolded as it had, while Ronald's was so different? How did it happen that two children born in the United States in the same year had come to have two such different lives? This was what I wondered as I lay in my bed in my room, thinking about him lying on that cot in his cell.

I referred earlier to the concept of otherness and the ways in which we divide ourselves into groups or camps: us and them. For reasons that are long-standing and complex, we human beings so often seem to fear the other (Ploesser & Mecheril, 2012). We fear that which is different. And we distance ourselves as much as possible from that which we fear. This distance takes us only to a place of greater misunderstanding where we know even less, and fear even more. If you take the time to think about it, you may find this pattern in your own experience as well. Ask yourself what it was that you learned about difference. Even if we were raised in an open and accepting family environment, the broader culture in which we are steeped is not always so generous. I have listened to people, especially the young, talk about growing up in towns that were largely homogenous, only to find that as they moved out into a more complex world, they didn't feel prepared for the diversity that they knew about intellectually, but had not experienced for themselves. Having said that, the path is not always so smooth in environments that are more diverse either.

When I was a boy, I grew up in Brooklyn in a neighborhood that had traditionally been populated most heavily by the Irish. There was a smattering of other ethnicities, however, including Norwegians and Germans. From my point of view as a boy, things seemed pretty easy going and peaceful, and the adult conversations I would listen in on confirmed that. As I approached adolescence, however, a change began to occur slowly in the neighborhood. Over time people began to speak of not walking down *that way*, not shopping on *that end* of the avenue. It just wasn't as nice. It was different, they said. After a while, I was able to pick up what the difference was; that part of the neighborhood was more and more home to a growing community of Hispanic immigrants—*them*.

Within a span of a few years, *their* territory had spread by quite a bit. The names on mailboxes and faces of people in the street had changed. Corner stores became bodegas with brightly lit signs advertising products that we had never heard of. A store-front church opened on my corner, and on hot summer nights, with the doors and windows thrown open and people sitting on their stoops, we could hear a music that was unfamiliar (particularly in the context of church), and the amplified sounds of people praising and worshipping.

All of this made a powerful impression not just on me, but also on the neighborhood as a whole. For some that impression was one of curiosity. For others, it grew into resentment. I remember hearing conversations among the adults wondering who *they* were and why *they* had come to our neighborhood. Why didn't they go back to where they came from or at least learn the language? Why didn't they learn how we did things here? Maybe some of that sounds familiar to you today? But there was an irony in all of this that I wasn't aware of until years later.

You see, when the ancestors of some of those very neighbors of ours arrived in the United States, most of them were Irish—*dirty Irish* as they were sometimes called back then. Along with the names came the judgments, stereotypes, and others forms of suspicion—all of which led to one conclusion. No one wanted the Irish around. So they were shoved off to a part of Brooklyn that was only beginning to develop, part of which was even still farmland. And an Irish ghetto was formed. Over the course of a few generations, that ghetto evolved into a lower middle class family neighborhood. By then, most people had long since forgotten their own roots—their own story.

So when the next wave of immigrants came in they too were greeted with suspicion and fear. They were most decidedly *"other."* The present generation had lost touch with its immigrant story, and the newly arrived were considered interlopers. Nevertheless, beyond the caricatures and stereotypes that were formed from initial experiences of difference, a deeper truth was there to be discovered. They were families, just like ours. Behind the veil of a language we could not speak, they were living lives that were not all that dissimilar from ours in their most important aspects—family, work, church, finding a community ….

If this tale sounds somewhat familiar to you, there is a good reason for that. It has been told in many ways, many times before. It is *West Side Story*, and its literary ancestor *Romeo and Juliet*. It is the story of those who get stuck on difference and who let their fear of the other balloon to sometimes epic proportions. It is a narrative that is enacted on playgrounds, in schools, and in the workplace. We encounter it among local communities and neighborhoods as well as larger racial and ethnic groups, and even nations as a whole (Baum, 2010).

Vamik Volkan (1988) has explored the ways in which, on levels from the individual to the international, we have a psychological need not only for allies but also for enemies. Enemies become the containers into which we can pour our fears, the screens onto which we can project the worst of our nature. This allows us to polarize each other, commonly viewing ourselves as "all good" and the other as "all bad" or something at least closely approximating that.

As social workers, when we encounter clients and communities that are torn by racial and ethnic strife, when we turn on the news and hear political spin in any direction about which lives matter, we need to be aware that narratives of *difference as threat* are at work. In those moments, as diplomats do in the international arena, we can bring to bear the powerful tools we have been discussing—our ability to see, to hear, and to empathize (as well as intervene) with the other who is before me. When we do so, we may be surprised to find out how often all the negative qualities we attribute to the racial and ethnic difference tie back to something else, something even deeper, and that is the evil of poverty.

Think about this in light of what we have been saying about the nature of social construction. In this instance we are talking about the relationship between race, ethnicity, and poverty and the social forces that undergird it. Begin with the concept of opportunity structures (Kirwan Institute, 2013). We know that economic, educational, health, and other developmental outcomes are highly related to environmental factors like adequate and affordable housing, stable employment that pays a living and hopefully growing wage, access to good schools, and quality health care and nutrition.

We also know that in environments where you find one of these, you are likely to find the others as well. Conversely, in neighborhoods, towns, cities, etc. where you find one of these lacking, the others are almost certainly lacking as well—or at the very least very hard to come by. The impact of this is to set up a system in which some have what might be referred to as a cumulative advantage while others have what we might call a cumulative disadvantage (Kirwan Institute, 2013). What we are talking about is, in effect, the structuralization of poverty. Some people refer here to the notion of intersectionality (Norris, Zajicek, & Murphy-Erby, 2010; Viruell-Fuentes, Miranda, & Abdulrahim, 2012), the theory that the impact of oppression along multiple lines (e.g., not only race but potentially also gender, sexual orientation, immigration status, mental health status, etc.) is not only additive, but also exponential. Intersectionality suggests that the burden of oppression becomes exponentially greater as more of these categories are added (Mattsson, 2014).

It will also likely not come as a surprise that the populations of communities impacted by cumulative disadvantage are disproportionately made up of racial and ethnic minorities (Corus et al., 2016; Quillian, 2012; Shuey & Wilson, 2008; Thoits, 2010). This in turn means that what we have come to think of as minority communities are also more highly impacted by the biopsychosocial outcomes associated with disadvantage. These include reduced life expectancy, compromised health and mental health, inadequate educational environments and higher dropout rates, limited job opportunities, and reduced income potential contributing to the intergenerational transmission of poverty. Related to this is multigenerational dependence on entitlement programs in the form of food, health care, and income subsidies. Interestingly, the theory of intersectionality has been criticized by some scholars interested in race who suggest that it may downplay the uniquely powerful role that racism has to play in the lives of people who are impacted by it (Hadden, Tolliver, Snowden, & Brown-Manning, 2016).

Additionally, we can consider a different but inextricably related layer of the social environment. In environments that are beset by so many dimensions of disadvantage we find a host of other outcomes as well. These include things like elevated levels of intimate partner violence, teen pregnancy, child abuse and neglect, and other forms of psychosocial trauma (King & Ogle, 2014). This inevitably makes environmental supports and life skills such as an adequate sense of emotional and physical safety, the ability to focus in school and to tolerate frustration, and the resilience to cope with adversity harder to come by (Eckenrode, Smith, McCarthy, & Dineen, 2014; Garmezy, 1991).

If we look further we find still more. All of these environmental challenges connected to poverty lead to disproportionate levels of alcohol and drug abuse (Mulia, Ye, Zemore, & Greenfield, 2008). In impoverished communities we find higher rates of crime and violence, and along with them, as in the case of Ronald, an increased likelihood of incarceration (Kutateladze, Andiloro, Johnson, & Spohn, 2014). What does it mean for us as a people, and what does it say about our social structures that half of the male African-American population of cities likes Baltimore are either incarcerated, on probation, or on parole?

At this point you might be thinking "All this is very interesting, even upsetting. But what does it have to do with narrative?" What I am suggesting is this. We have socially constructed institutions and other environmental forces that have led to the marginalization of communities of racial and ethnic minorities. We have created social structures that set up and reinforce conditions of poverty in these same communities. When the almost inevitable outcomes of poverty then arise, we create a communal narrative that blames the poor for these outcomes. Not only that, we spin the tale that these outcomes—drug abuse, crime, violence, dependence on public assistance … are the by-products of race and ethnicity, not poverty. We create a climate that alienates those who are different as "other" in ways that breed at best suspicion, and at worst outright fear and aggression.

Perhaps nowhere is this better seen than in the criminal justice system. We must ask what are the social forces that underlie the hugely disproportionate number of African-Americans incarcerated in the United States (Alexander, 2012). While African-Americans make up only 13% of the population in the United States, they represent over 40% of people incarcerated (U.S. Census Bureau, 2015 as cited in Hadden et al., 2016). People like Bryan Stevenson (2014) and Michelle Alexander (2012) have taken up as a calling the imperative to shed light on the socially constructed forces that are behind the demonization (together with incarceration and even execution) of the other particularly in the form of race and ethnicity. Even outside of the corrections system per se, narratives of difference around race underlie conflicts between police and communities of color. In these conflicts, young black men are often perceived as inherently dangerous and thus the targets of aggression by law enforcement (Aymer, 2016). Some might respond to this, "But it isn't simply a story. There *is* greater violence in many minority communities. There *is* greater drug use and gang activity." My goal here is not to dispute crime statistics. It is to consider the nature of the socially constructed forces that undergird those statistics and that conspire to keep systemic disadvantage and marginalization in place. Key among these, I am suggesting, is the kind of projection that Volkan (1988) speaks of, the force that allows us to marginalize the other along the lines of race and ethnicity and that creates the kind of poverty structure that is so difficult to dismantle because it is so pervasive and so socially reinforced. Moskowitz (1995) makes this point as well, noting that ethnicity and race are fantasies that we can use to project our sense of badness onto the other.

The social structures that keep the poverty-generating forces of marginalization in place are so insidious not only as to be easy to miss, but also as to be easy to internalize. Members of communities that are beset by the crime and violence that stem from systemic disadvantage may find themselves identified with the negative projections cast upon them. This may be manifested as a sense of self and community in which they see themselves as "less than." The experience of disenfranchisement may be so great as to quash the ability to hope and to limit the horizon of the future to more of the same. Consider, for example, findings that suggest that, regardless of the data pertaining to actual income, individuals who self-identify as black are less likely to consider themselves members of the middle or upper class (Speer, 2016). In other words, actual income does not necessarily relate to the sense of self when it comes to class position. Speer (2016) goes on to suggest that this discrepancy is related to experience of discrimination and inequality.

Related to this are within-group manifestations of racial and ethnic bias. These may be expressed as a preference for or the favorability of individuals of a certain skin tone or hair texture, for example. It may be internalized in the form of a negative self-image related to these same qualities. A young African-American woman I worked with for several years consistently felt negatively compared to her sister, and compared herself negatively as well. Unable to see how attractive she was or to take ownership of her considerable professional success, she believed that her family, and the world for that matter, favored her sister because she had lighter skin and straighter hair. This phenomenon is also extended to ethnic groups such as when Latinos from one country hold and promote negative stereotypes of individuals from other countries.

The correlate of these dynamics of marginalization that we have been discussing is the related construct of white privilege (McIntosh, 1998, 2015). This is almost certainly a concept you have explored in some depth in social work school—the notion that just as racial and ethnic minorities have been disadvantaged in pervasive, systematic ways, so too have white people been privileged. This is challenging for many to see, of course, since from the perspective of our Caucasian-dominated master narrative, white people are largely accustomed to viewing this not as a systematic and socially constructed advantage, but simply the way things are. I have heard people, learning about the notion of white privilege, retort, "Well that doesn't make any sense. I never asked for any privilege and I have had struggles too." This, of course, misses the point. I recall hearing a lecture on white privilege many years ago in which the speaker, a white woman in her early 30s, apologized profusely for her whiteness and the way it had negatively impacted many others. However sincere that young woman was in delivering her lecture, it came across as painfully awkward.

It goes without saying that all people struggle and even encounter disadvantage in ways that may have a truly adverse impact. It is also fairly clear, I hope, that no one need to apologize for the color of the skin or the racial and ethnic heritage into which they were born. What is important, however, for the sake of justice, is the acknowledgement that socially constructed forces, long-standing and with roots deeply planted in a history of division and oppression, do work together for the systematic advantage of some and the disadvantage of others. These forces do predict that the horizon is set higher for some than others. They do bring with them statistically predictable differences in overall educational attainment, health and mental health status and outcome, teen pregnancy, likelihood of incarceration, and even life expectancy. I am suggesting that the best first step in responding to white privilege is to acknowledge it and the ways in which some benefit from it while others are oppressed by it. This offers us the opportunity to work together to address it, correct it, and pursue a deeper form of justice.

It is also important for us to address another phenomenon that occurs with respect to race and ethnicity and may even flow from the dynamics of white privilege that we have been discussing, and that is the microaggression (Owen, Tao, Imel, Wampold, & Rodolfa, 2014). This too is likely something that you have discussed in your social work classes, perhaps particularly any course you have taken related to diversity. Microaggressions are another manifestation of implicit bias (Kirwan Institute, 2016). However, these are not expressed with the negative valence that is typical and expected when it comes to matters of race and ethnicity. They may even have an emotional tone that feels superficially positive. But therein lies the problem.

Microaggressions are manifested in at least a couple of different ways. They may seek to express something positive, a compliment of sorts, to the receiver, not based on an attribute of that individual specifically, but rather a generalized quality that is laid upon the person based on their race or ethnicity. You have no doubt heard such comments, whether or not you knew that you could call them microaggressions. This occurs, for example, when a person of Asian ancestry is told, "Oh, you must be so smart." Or "You're probably really good at math and science." It is expressed when people suggest things like "African Americans are such great athletes." Again, note that the emotional valence of these kinds of statements is at least superficially positive or complimentary. They are likely intended, in some sort of unexamined way, to express praise for the recipient. In spite of this, they are expressions of bias that are based on racial and ethnic stereotypes.

Another kind of microaggression comes in the denial of being impacted by bias. The kinds of processes that we have been discussing, this predilection for categorization, and then judgment based on perceived categories are ubiquitous in human society. All of us have been touched in some way by the bias implicit in stereotypes of all kinds. We are all aware on some level of difference. Occasionally you might hear a person say something like "Race and ethnicity don't matter to me. I don't see color. I don't see difference." While this may be well intentioned and may even correspond to a good deal of nonjudgmental acceptance of difference on the part of that individual, I would suggest that it is nonetheless naïve. Each of us is aware of difference, the *other*—whether that otherness is attributed to someone else or even ourselves.

There is yet another facet to this, however. My identity, and sense of self and place in the world, is also intimately tied to my experience of affiliation/disaffiliation with a racial and ethnic heritage. They are not by any means the sum total of who I am, but they are a part of my story. And so to tell another human being that I don't see color and that I don't see difference is to say that I don't see you. It strips away the opportunity to listen and learn from you about that dimension of your identity and experience. It deprives both of us of the possibility of fostering the genuine connection that can come not from the illusion of sameness but the acknowledgement, even with all of its challenges, of the gift of difference.

While it may seem to some that I have been describing issues more commonly associated with macro social work practice, all of this matters deeply to us as clinicians. When we enter the room with a client, among the many powerful things that are beginning to occur is this. That client brings with him or her all of who they are—everything that has shaped them as persons up to that point. And of course, the same can be said for us—whoever we are. We enter that space together having been formed by the social and cultural forces around us. So when we enter that room, whether we speak of it or not, race and ethnicity enter that room. I would even go so far as to suggest to you that race and ethnicity are in that room even when we imagine that the other person, be it client or therapist, is "someone like me." In fact, this kind of assumption may at times be even more insidious if the lack of apparent difference seduces us into believing that we must be the same. While the impressions and assumptions of our clients are always grist for the mill, as they say, we as social workers need to be ever mindful of the dynamics of difference, whether that difference is visible or not. What we see before our eyes may not correspond to the sense of self of the other when it comes to difference or similarity (Mendez, 2015).

Let me give you an example. I once attended a supervision training course given by a respected social worker whose name I knew, but whom I had never met. It so happens that she is Caucasian. One of the earliest topics that was covered was culture and its impact on supervision. She told this story. When she was a girl, her parents were both Christian missionaries. They lived and worked in Africa, which was where she was born and raised. As happens in one's native land, she knew and felt herself to be at home. Though she was racially in the minority, the world around her did not feel alien. It was hers—the people, the culture, the sounds, the food, and the customs—all hers. When she was older, she moved to the United States with her parents, Americans by birth. It was here that she began to have an experience of difference. When she arrived in New Jersey, to a predominantly Caucasian environment, she noticed how she blended in and how, because of the color of her skin, the social and cultural world around her took her in as one of their own. The irony, however, was that she experienced herself very much as a foreigner. She described how she felt and continued to feel much more of a sense of belonging among people from Africa—no matter how she appeared on the outside.

When we come together in a therapeutic space with a client of whatever race or ethnicity, it is essential that we acknowledge and allow their stories and ours to be with us in the room. We may make a clinical choice not to share much of our own story, but we must be aware of what it is and be attentive to its potential influence in our work. So just how do we go about this? I'm going to suggest something that you might find both simple and challenging: ask. As I said in Chap. 1, wonder with your client. Invite them to share their experience. To begin with, we might ask our clients to tell us how *they* identify their race or ethnicity, even if they had to check a box on the demographic section of an intake form. This is a foundational piece of this part of their narrative. It is theirs to name, not ours to infer by appearance or accent or any other outward sign that we might interpret correctly or incorrectly. So it absolutely matters whether a person identifies as black or African-American, African, or Afro-Caribbean. It matters deeply if their ancestors came from the American South or South Africa.

It so happens that I speak Spanish fluently and have spent the majority of my adult life living and working in the Latino world. Many years ago, I was living and working in the South Bronx and was invited to give a series of workshops at a church in an almost entirely Caucasian suburb. One of the local leaders was asking about my work. As I shared some of the struggles that my largely Puerto Rican and Dominican community was having, he smiled and said,

> "Well at least they have all of that wonderful mariachi music!"
> A bit taken aback, I replied, "Well no. Mariachi music is Mexican."
> "Isn't it all the same?" he asked.

No. It is most decidedly not all the same. And it matters deeply whether a person identifies as Puerto Rican or Dominican, or Colombian, Peruvian, Salvadoran, Mexican, and so on …. It most decidedly matters if someone identifies as Chinese, Japanese, Korean, Thai, or Filipino. And while we're at it, it matters, often deeply, whether a person identifies as Italian, Irish, Norwegian, or Moldovan. It also matters *how much* it matters to them. How important is that sense of racial or ethnic identity? If they are members of an immigrant family, how long have they been in the United States? What has their process of acculturation been like? What is the role of their race or ethnicity in their family narrative?

Imagine what it would be like, as you are gathering all of the clinical information that we do from a client to ask something like "Can you share with me how you feel your experience has been shaped by your race (or ethnic identity)?" Imagine using that respectful wondering to ask what if any experience they have had with racism or discrimination.

Then imagine asking how they experience being there with you, and the prospect of working with you. The intake should not be the only time these issues are addressed. They should be attended to as needed throughout the course of our work together since they will continue to have an impact on the narrative we are crafting together in treatment. However, it is important in my view that we set a tone in that first meeting by addressing difference, by wondering about it with the client. In this way, we take the burden off the client who may or may not be thinking about it, and who might be concerned that it would be inappropriate to mention. We signal to them that we are aware of it and offer it as a potentially important dimension of experience to explore. We also communicate that, even if the topic is an emotionally charged one, we can handle it together (Candelario & Huber, 2002).

Having mentioned this notion of taking the burden off the client let me say that it is equally important that we attend to the dynamics of power in the room. There is of course already a power differential when one person occupies the position of client and the other the position of therapist. In therapeutic dyads in which the client is of a minority background and the therapist of majority background, this may be especially important to be aware of and to address (Chang & Berk, 2009; Chang & Yoon, 2011). If therapist and client are of the same ancestry or at least share an identification as belonging to a racial or ethnic minority, the power differential may manifest around perceptions of educational attainment, social class, or some other category.

I have advocated for a stance of curiosity, or wondering. Let me mention another way in which I believe this is important when it comes to race and ethnicity, and other dimensions of difference as well. As social workers we must be attentive for any ways we find ourselves presuming what a client will think, feel, or prefer. For example, I have heard social workers say things like "Well she's a young woman so she would probably be most comfortable working with a woman." or "Men are going to have an easier time opening up to another man." We may assume that clients will be most comfortable with a therapist whom *we perceive* to be most like them. And we may be dead wrong. In the end, then, don't assume. Wonder.

Case Example

It was a rainy Tuesday afternoon when Yolanda arrived at the mental health clinic about a mile from her apartment for an intake. She had called the week before asking to see someone. She spoke little English so she required a Spanish-speaking therapist. But she went further, requesting to be seen by a female who was also Latina. There was one person on the staff who met that description, an excellent therapist who would have been wonderful for Yolanda. As it happened though, the therapist she was scheduled to see was sick that day and had called out of the office. I had an opening on my calendar, and the secretary asked if I would at least do the intake.

When I greeted Yolanda in the waiting room she was understandably confused and appeared uncomfortable. Though I was speaking Spanish, I was clearly not the person she had been expecting. Not wanting to discuss the situation in front of the other clients who were waiting, I asked if we could go back to my office for a moment to talk so that I could explain the situation. She agreed and followed me down the hall. When we sat down, I explained that, unfortunately, the therapist she was scheduled to see was sick that day and wasn't in the office. In an effort to reassure her and acknowledge that she was in charge of her treatment, I offered her a couple of options. I told her that we could simply reschedule the appointment with the therapist for another day and she could return. If she was willing, however, I told her that I also had time to meet with her. If she liked I could at least conduct an initial intake as a way of getting the ball rolling. If she still wanted to see the other therapist after we had finished, I would be more than happy to schedule that and to pass on everything she shared with me to the other therapist. Yolanda paused for a moment to consider her options and reluctantly said that she would stay for the appointment and talk to me this one time. I told her that was more than fine.

I learned that Yolanda was a 32-year-old single mother of three girls aged 16, 15, and 12. She and her children lived in a small apartment in the inner city neighborhood surrounding the clinic. She had come to that city from her native Dominican Republic when she was in her early 20s. Yolanda did not work and had no substantial work history; she had briefly held jobs in a couple of local factories, but not in several years. In fact, it turned out, Yolanda rarely left her apartment, relying on her children and sometimes her boyfriend who visited regularly to buy groceries and run errands. On that day, her 16-year-old daughter, who was out in the waiting room, accompanied her to the clinic.

Yolanda initially attributed her difficulty leaving the house, even coming to the clinic on her own, to the discomfort she felt being outside alone. As we proceeded, Yolanda shared with me a story of profound trauma. Though not able to go into great detail, she told me that her father sexually abused her from the ages of 13–16. When her parents divorced and her mother remarried, she hoped that the abuse would stop. However, he would arrange for times to be alone with her, often going to great lengths to do so, and the abuse continued. The abuse only ended when she left her mother's home at 16 to marry her then boyfriend. She dropped out of high school and soon had her first child. Though she knew that her father had died several years previously, she told me that she still felt he was there, that he was continuing to persecute her.

As we continued to talk, Yolanda described for me a host of symptoms of depression and anxiety. I also heard clearly in her description the presence of almost every symptom of post-traumatic stress disorder. Her trauma was so severe that at times it disrupted her reality testing. These moments were terrifying for her. Yolanda's voice was soft, often like a whisper. Her eye contact was poor and her affect flat. She was neatly dressed and well groomed. Though she was a tall woman and somewhat overweight, she appeared delicate and fragile. Yolanda had been in treatment a couple of times in the past, but she had a hard time sticking with therapy. She had felt that no one understood (an indirect communication about what she was looking for and needed in a therapist). One therapist, cherry-picking some of her more sensational symptoms while missing the broad picture entirely, had even diagnosed her with schizophrenia.

As we came to the end of that initial interview, I shared some impressions with Yolanda, careful to acknowledge that she had only recounted what I was sure was the smallest fraction of her story. I told her that I could hear the trauma she had endured, and offered that, in my view, everything that she had and was continuing to experience fit into the narrative of a person who was wounded in that way. Though I was easily able to see myself working with Yolanda, I was also aware that she had expressed a preference for working with my Latina colleague. I asked Yolanda what she thought she would like to do—reiterating that she was entirely in control of the decision and that whatever she chose was perfectly fine. I went so far as to tell her sincerely that the Latina therapist whom she was scheduled to see was perhaps the best therapist I knew. To my surprise, Yolanda said with only slight hesitation that she thought she would like to come back and see me. We scheduled another appointment and she left. Yolanda and I wound up working together for over 4 years, much of it on a twice-a-week basis.

As you might imagine, Yolanda's therapy was at times intense and even painful. There were sessions in which all we could do was work on containment. At other times we had to focus on helping her manage the day-to-day business of life, complicated not only by her economic struggle and inability to speak much English, but also by the fact that she had such difficulty leaving her house. We did of course work together, slowly and patiently, on healing the trauma she endured.

Even beyond the experience of actual sexual abuse, she spoke of the ways her father had terrorized her psychologically. While she lived in the Dominican Republic, her father had moved to the mainland United States. She prayed that his move would bring an end to the abuse, and it did slow down. But in a way that was almost more psychologically cruel, her father would show up at her home at random times wanting to see her. He would travel to the Dominican Republic unexpectedly and Yolanda, arriving home from school, would find him sitting in the living room of the home she shared with her mother and stepfather, waiting for her. On those occasions, he would typically take her out to spend some time with her, and would abuse her once again. She recounted his admonitions never to tell her mother or stepfather what was happening between them, assuring her that he could and would kill them all in their sleep.

Yolanda also shared with me concerns that she had about her boyfriend, a Puerto Rican man named Raul, and the conflicted feelings she had about their relationship. On the one hand, she depended on him. Raul gave her some money and often brought groceries to the apartment. She thought it was important, even for her children, to have a man around the house, but didn't like the way he would show up unexpectedly and try to take charge, telling the children what to do—even just randomly changing the T.V. channel as he occupied his favorite chair.

His visits seemed random. Because of Yolanda's struggles they did not go out on traditional dates or even run errands together. He might go days and even a week or more without visiting. She began to feel that he only came around when he wanted sex—something that almost always happened regardless of whether Yolanda was in the mood or not. Raul never slept in the apartment. When the sex was over, he would leave. Yolanda strongly suspected that he had other women, perhaps even a genuine relationship, on the side. But she had no way of proving it, and Raul denied it.

One afternoon, after we had been working together for about a year, Yolanda came to session and said that she would like to talk about something new that she had begun to notice. She told me that she had been experiencing intense fears for her youngest daughter, Jennifer. She worried about her walking to and from school. She worried about her being all right when she was in school. She worried that someone might harm her every time she left the house, even if she was with one of her elder sisters. She worried that someone—a man—might harm her, take her, and abuse her. Recently, Yolanda arrived home with her eldest daughter from an appointment and found Raul in the apartment alone with Jennifer. She became furious with him, demanding to know what was going on and why he was there. Both Raul and Jennifer seemed confused by her anger. Yolanda said that she had no idea where these fears came from or why she was concerned about Jennifer in particular.

Yolanda and I explored these feelings of fear. We did our best to look at their content as well as moments when they arose, and wondered together about what brought them on. I asked Yolanda if she recalled ever having similar fears for her two elder daughters. She thought about it briefly and said yes; as a matter of fact she had experienced the same fears for both of her other daughters, but no longer did. Yolanda thought that was curious, and I could see on her face that she was trying to make sense of the story of how these fears came and went. She intuited, as did I, that her fears were not only related to the story she was telling herself about Jennifer or her other children for that matter, but also about herself and her own experiences as well. So we tried to understand Yolanda's concerns in the context of her narrative, her story of herself as a girl and now a woman, as well as the men who had been significant in her life—the father who abused her, the ex-husband who had left her, and the boyfriend who reminded her in so many ways of her father. Yolanda had a consuming story of her vulnerability as a woman and the abusive intent of men.

The more Yolanda and I sat with and explored the dynamics of this narrative, the more we were able to understand her current concerns for Jennifer and her past concerns for her other daughters. What we discovered was that this fear of her daughters being abused by men surfaced when they reached the age of 13—that age at which she herself was first abused. Yolanda similarly realized that her fears dissipated when they turned 16, the age at which she left the house to get married and was freed from the grip of her abusive father. Yolanda understood that an unarticulated part of her narrative up to that point was that the onset of the teen years was a time of heightened vulnerability for her daughters and in fact, she thought, for all girls. Sixteen, however, represented an age of freedom and independence. It was a time when a young woman could take greater control of her life and be more vigilant for her own safety. This was a terribly important insight for Yolanda. Though it did not dispel all of her fears, understanding the meaning of this part of her narrative allowed her a greater measure of peace and control over them.

In spite of what I recommended earlier, I will confess that Yolanda and I, now working together for some time, had not yet spoken of the apparent differences between us. Yet, if you are paying attention and open to it, these things do have a way of surfacing even all on their own. Yolanda arrived for her appointment one day and began by commenting that she thought she knew which car in the large municipal parking lot outside was mine. She noticed it there, amidst more than a hundred other cars mind you, every time she came to see me. I asked Yolanda which one it was and she said, "It's the silver Jaguar."

There are many ways to look at this moment from a therapeutic point of view, but what I was interested in was understanding the narrative that I knew had been forming in Yolanda's mind. We had worked together in therapy closely for quite some time, and I knew that she was bonded to me. I even suspected, though we had not gotten to explore it yet, that she had strong feelings for me. As is common for many therapists, the default position that I consistently adopt in therapy is one of relative anonymity. In other words, I share very little if anything about my own life and myself. So I felt that this was an important therapeutic opportunity.

> "What is it that makes you believe the silver Jaguar is mine?"
> "I don't know. I think it's just the kind of car someone like you would drive," she said thoughtfully.
> "Someone like me? Tell me more. What is it about that car? What is it about me?"
> "The Jaguar is for someone who is smart and successful. It's powerful."
> "So, is that how you think and feel about me? Smart, successful, powerful?"
> "Well…yeah," she offered timidly. "I hope that's ok. Have I offended you?"
> "No. Not at all," I reassured her. "I think you're talking about something really important, and I find myself wondering how that impression affects the way you relate to me."

The narrative that unfolded as Yolanda spoke revealed not only what she thought of me, but also what she thought about herself and how she experienced the perceived difference between us. The story she had constructed about my life suggested her idealization of me, and her sense that our lives bore nothing in common whatsoever. Yolanda imagined that I was a person of considerable wealth who lived in an exclusive neighborhood in a beautiful house, my silver Jaguar parked in my spacious garage. I could have anything and do anything I wanted. Yolanda went on to describe her fantasy about my wife and how she fit into this narrative. In her imagination, my wife was a tall, thin blonde woman. She was a businesswoman who dressed in expensive suits and worked in New York City. She always wore her hair in a tight bun, and had an air about her that Yolanda described as "severe." She was strong and tough.

By contrast, Yolanda then described herself as poor, troubled, uneducated, overweight, and unattractive. She found it hard to name any of her many positive qualities, even when prompted. She felt damaged and undesirable. Her life had been populated with men who were disappointing at best and brutally destructive at worst. She didn't imagine that her lot would change very much. Revealing even more of her countertransference she said, "A man like you would never have any interest in a woman like me." In Yolanda's narrative, the fact that I worked at the mental health clinic was evidence that I was an exceptionally good person, since I would be willing to step away from my comfortable life and "come help people like her." I had even gone to the trouble of learning Spanish so that I could use it in my work. She was pleased that I had taken a professional interest in people like her and was willing to learn something about her and her culture so that I could try to help.

I invite you to take a moment and sit with this narrative. It is a story of parallel lives in parallel worlds—lives and worlds that were completely different except for the fact that I would choose to step out of my world in the course of the workday and step into hers. As bonded as Yolanda felt to me, her story revealed to me her sense that this white man of privilege could never really understand a poor Latina like herself. I echoed this back to her and she confirmed, almost apologetically, that she did in fact feel this way.

At this point I was contemplating and ultimately chose to use self-disclosure in a way that was uncharacteristic of me and that I felt uncertain of even as I was doing it. It is not something I would recommend to a beginning therapist without first discussing it with a good supervisor. I began by telling Yolanda that I felt like there were a couple of things that I wanted to share with her. First, I too had seen the silver Jaguar in the parking lot. It was there most days of the week, but it wasn't in fact mine. I told her that my car was actually 10 years old. I did not reveal the make or model, as I didn't want to encourage her to going looking for it.

Then I went further. I chose to share with Yolanda that my wife is, in fact, Latina herself. Yolanda was visibly stunned. She paused for a moment, and then wondered if she could ask me a couple of questions. I agreed.

"What country is she from?"
"Costa Rica. She was born there, but came here when she was young."
"Does she speak Spanish?"
"Yes."
"Do you ever speak Spanish with her… at home…?"
"Sure. We speak English most of the time, but often speak in Spanish. Her parents don't speak much English so when they're around we only speak Spanish."
"Do you ever eat Latin food? (something of a poor translation of the Spanish phrase)."
"Yeah. All the time."
She paused, processing this.

I told Yolanda that I was wondering what she was thinking and feeling, what all of this meant to her.

After a moment, she said, "Two things. One is that I like knowing that speaking Spanish isn't just part of your job. It's part of your real life; I never imagined that." She hesitated.

"What's the second thing?" I asked.

"It means that you might really understand me. You know something about Latinas, not just from books, but for real."

We both laughed.

"That's true. I do know something about Latinas, at least some of them," I said.

"It means something else too," she added.

"What's that?"

"I guess I never thought that a man like you could be interested in a woman like me."

This exchange with her felt uncommonly rich, and perhaps in another context we could start to unpack all of the layers of meaning in it. For our purposes, however, my hope is that you will tune into the dimension of this story that is most pertinent for the discussion we have been having. Yolanda and I each brought to our therapeutic relationship a different, and until that day unspoken, story about what our ethnic (and other) differences meant. There were issues of power, class, and perceived potential. But for Yolanda it was all wrapped up in the ethnic and cultural differences between us, and the way those were embodied in the symbol of language.

We were of course different in many ways. Consistent with what we explored earlier, Yolanda's life and opportunities were very much impacted by poverty. It affected her finances, her education, her access to health care, and more. She was also painfully wounded by the trauma she had endured. Nonetheless, something about our exchange that day forged a bridge, a different kind of understanding between us that helped facilitate the work we continued to do together for over two more years.

It does not escape my attention that someone reading this might think that there's something neat and tidy about this story. It worked out really well. But what if it wasn't so neat? What if my wife weren't Latina and we didn't speak Spanish at home. What if I didn't particularly enjoy Spanish food? What if the silver Jaguar were in fact mine? What would I do then? These are all excellent and important questions, and ones that I have contemplated over the years since I knew Yolanda. The truth is this. I don't entirely know. But I can tell you what I hope.

The story I shared with you unfolded as it did because Yolanda and I created a space that day in which she could reveal something more about her story and, because it felt appropriate to do so in that context, I chose to reveal something more about mine. (Note that I did not go into great detail about my life. As always, it was essential to keep the focus on Yolanda, and I only chose to share some information that I felt would be meaningful to her story and the story we were constructing together.) If the facts of my life had been different, I hope that my goal would have been the same—to be open, to listen, to understand as best I can, and to be as genuine as possible. The outcome would be unique, because the stories of our clients and the evolution of those stories that we are privileged to witness and to co-construct are always unique. There is evidence that suggests that in therapy with a mixed racial or ethnic dyad of therapist and client, a key factor is the client's awareness of the therapist's desire to understand and help the client pursue their goals. Similarly, the ability to acknowledge and work through ruptures and challenges to the relationship is invaluable (Chang & Berk, 2009; Chang & Yoon, 2011).

Race and ethnicity are in the room with us because they are part of who we all are. No matter how different or similar we think we are or appear to be, our work remains the same. As we explore the meaning of race and ethnicity for our clients as well as for ourselves, we open up new possibilities of growth, understanding, and healing of that important part of our narrative.

Questions and Activities for Discussion and Further Reflection

1. Reflect on your own story of race and ethnicity. Consider your own family ancestry and the extent to which race and ethnicity have been important aspects of your own identity. Have you had any experiences or racism or other forms of discrimination? If so, how have these contributed to the shaping of your own narrative with respect to race and ethnicity?
2. What experiences have you had with difference in your life? How close has difference come to your personal life? What feelings are elicited by difference (e.g., interest, excitement, disorientation, fear)? How has that shaped your own story?
3. How comfortable or uncomfortable do you imagine you would be addressing issues of race and ethnicity with a client? What is it about yourself or the topic that might lead you to feel that way?
4. Engage in a class discussion about the social construction of race and ethnicity and the implications that has for identity development for each of us. Search for ways in which socially constructed narratives of race and ethnicity are presented in the culture (e.g., through media). Share these with each other as well as your own reactions to them.
5. Search through recent news and other media for information about what people of different backgrounds are saying about racism and ethnic discrimination. Keeping in mind what you have learned in this chapter about narratives of race and ethnicity, what do you understand about the factors that have shaped the stories behind these different perspectives?
6. Did any of the examples or stories in this chapter stand out to you in particular? If so, which ones? What in particular struck you about that narrative? Does it suggest anything to you about your own story or that of your clients?
7. Articulate for yourself your understanding of the most important factors for a social worker to keep when trying to attend to the narrative of race or ethnicity of his or her clients?

References

Alexander, M. (2012). *The new Jim Crow: Mass incarceration in the age of colorblindness*. New York: The New Press.
Aymer, S. R. (2016). "I can't breathe": A case study—helping black men cope with race-related trauma stemming from police killing and brutality. *Journal of Human Behavior in the Social Environment*, 26(3–4), 367–376.

Baum, N. (2010). After a terror attack: Israeli—Arab professionals' feelings and experiences. *Journal of Social and Personal Relationships, 27*(5), 685–704. https://doi.org/10.1177/0265407510368965

Baum, N. (2011). Issues in psychotherapy with clients affiliated with the opposing side in a violenct political conflict. *Clinical Social Work Journal, 39*, 91–100.

Candelario, N., & Huber, H. (2002). A school-based experience on racial identity and race relations. *Smith College Studies in Social Work, 73*(1), 51–72.

Chang, D. F., & Berk, A. (2009). Making cross-racial therapy work: A phenomenological study of clients' experiences of cross-racial therapy. *Journal of Counseling Psychology, 56*(4), 521–536.

Chang, D. F., & Yoon, P. (2011). Ethnic minority clients' perceptions of the significance of race in cross-racial therapy relationships. *Psychotherapy Research, 21*(5), 567–582. https://doi.org/10.1080/10503307.2011.592549

Corus, C., Saatcioglu, B., Kaufman-Scarborough, C., Blocker, C. P., Upadhyaya, S., & Appau, S. (2016). Transforming poverty-related policy with intersectionality. *Journal of Public Policy and Marketing, 35*(2), 211–222.

Eckenrode, J., Smith, E. G., McCarthy, M. E., & Dineen, M. (2014). Income inequality and child maltreatment in the United States. *Pediatrics, 133*(3), 454–461. https://doi.org/10.1542/peds.2013-1707

Garmezy, N. (1991). Resiliency and vulnerability to adverse developmental outcomes associated with poverty. *American Behavioral Scientist, 34*(4), 416–430.

Godley, A. J., & Loretto, A. (2013). Fostering counter-narratives of race, language, and identity in an urban English classroom. *Linguistics and Education, 24*, 316–327.

Gomez, L. E. (2012). Looking for race in all the wrong places. *Law & Society Review, 46*(2), 221–245.

Hadden, B. R., Tolliver, W., Snowden, F., & Brown-Manning, R. (2016). An authentic discourse: Recentering race and racism as factors that contribute to police violence against unarmed black or african american men. *Journal of Human Behavior in the Social Environment, 26*(3–4), 336–349.

Hill, M. R., & Thomas, V. (2000). Strategies for racial identity development: Narratives of black and white women in interracial partner relationships. *Family Relations, 49*(2), 193–200.

Keddell, E. (2009). Narrative as identity: Postmodernism, multiple ethnicities, and narrative practice approaches in social work. *Journal of Ethnic and Cultural Diversity in Social Work, 18*(3), 221–241.

King, K., & Ogle, C. (2014). Negative life events vary by neighborhood and mediate the relation between neighborhood context and psychological well-being. *PLoS One, 9*(4), e93539. https://doi.org/10.1371/journal.pone.0093539

Kirwan Institute. (2013). *Structural racialization: A systems approach to understanding the causes and consequences of racial inequality*. Retrieved from http://kirwaninstitute.osu.edu/docs/NewSR-brochure-FINAL.pdf.

Kirwan Institute. (2016). *State of the science: Implicit bias review*. Retrieved from http://kirwaninstitute.osu.edu/my-product/2016-state-of-the-science-implicit-bias-review/.

Kutateladze, B. L., Andiloro, N. R., Johnson, B. D., & Spohn, C. C. (2014). Cumulative disadvantage: Examining racial and ethnic disparity in prosecution and sentencing. *Criminology, 52*(3), 514–551. https://doi.org/10.1111/1745-9125.12047

Lawrence, C. (2012). Listening for stories in all the right places: Narratives and racial formation theory. *Law & Society Review, 46*(2), 247–258.

Mattsson, T. (2014). Intersectionality as a useful tool: Anti-oppressive social work and critical reflection. *Affilia, 29*(1), 8–17.

McIntosh, P. (1998). White privilege: Unpacking the invisible knapsack. In M. McGoldrick (Ed.), *Re-visioning family therapy: Race, culture, and gender in clinical practice* (pp. 147–152). New York, NY: Guilford Press.

McIntosh, P. (2015). Extending the knapsack: Using the white privilege analysis to examine conferred advantage and disadvantage. *Women & Therapy, 38*(3–4), 232–245. https://doi.org/10.1080/02703149.2015.1059195

References

Mendez, T. (2015). "My sister tried to kill me": Enactment and foreclosure in a mixed-race dyad. *Psychodyn Psychiatry, 43*(2), 229–242.

Moskowitz, M. (1995). Ethnicity and the fantasy of ethnicity. *Psychoanalytic Psychology, 12*(4), 547–555. https://doi.org/10.1037/h0079690

Mulia, N., Ye, Y., Zemore, S. E., & Greenfield, T. K. (2008). Social disadvantage, stress, and alcohol use among Black, Hispanic, and White Americans: Findings from the 2005 U.S. National Alcohol Survey. *Journal of Studies on Alcohol and Drugs, 69*(6), 824–833. 10.15288/jsad.2008.69.824

Norris, A. N., Zajicek, A., & Murphy-Erby, Y. (2010). Intersectional perspective and rural poverty research: Benefits, challenges and policy implications. *Journal of Poverty, 14*(1), 55–75. https://doi.org/10.1080/10875540903489413

Nuttman-Shwartz, O. (2008). *Working with "others": In a context of political conflict, is it possible to support clients whose views you disagree with? Manuscript.*

Owen, J., Tao, K. W., Imel, Z., Wampold, B. E., & Rodolfa, E. (2014). Addressing racial and ethnic microaggressions in therapy. *Professional Psychology: Research and Practice, 45*(4), 283–290.

Ploesser, M., & Mecheril, P. (2012). Neglect—recognition—destruction: Approaches to otherness in social work. *International Social Work, 55*(6), 794–808.

Polkinghorne, D. E. (1988). *Narrative knowing and the human sciences*. Alban, NY: State University of New York Press.

Pyne, K. B., & Means, D. R. (2013). Underrepresented and in/visible: A Hispanic first-generation student's narratives of college. *Journal of Diversity in Higher Education, 6*(3), 186–198.

Quillian, L. (2012). Segregation and poverty concentration: The role of three segregations. *American Sociological Review, 77*(3), 354–379.

Rockquemore, K. A., & Laszloffy, T. A. (2003). Multiple realities: A relational narrative approach in therapy with black-white-mixed-race clients. *Family Relations, 52*(2), 119–128.

Shuey, K. M., & Wilson, A. E. (2008). Cumulative disadvantage and black-white disparities in life-course health trajectories. *Research on Aging, 30*(2), 200–225.

Smedley, A., & Smedley, B. D. (2005). Race as biology is fiction, racism as social problem is real. *American Psychologist, 60*(1), 16–26.

Speer, I. (2016). Race, wealth and class identification in 21st-century american society. *The Sociological Quarterly, 57*, 356–379.

Stevenson, B. (2014). *Just mercy: A story of justice and redemption*. New York: Spiegel & Grau.

Stonequest, E. (1935). The problem of the marginal man. *American Journal of Sociology, 41*, 1–12.

Sue, D. W., & Sue, D. (2016). *Counseling the culturally diverse: Theory and practice* (7th ed.). Hoboken: Wiley.

Thoits, P. A. (2010). Stress and health: Major findings and policy implications. *Journal of Health and Social Behavior, 51*(1), S41–S53.

U.S. Census Bureau. (2015). *State and county quickfacts. Data derived from population estimates, American community survey, census of population and housing, state and county housing unit estimates, county business patterns, non-employer statistics, economic census, survey of business owners, building permits*. Retrieved from http://quickfacts.census.gov/qfd/states/00000.html.

Viruell-Fuentes, E. A., Miranda, P. Y., & Abdulrahim, S. (2012). More than culture: Structural racism, intersectionality theory, and immigrant health. *Social Science & Medicine, 75*(12), 2099–2106. https://doi.org/10.1016/j.socscimed.2011.12.037

Volkan, V. (1988). *The need to have enemies and allies: From clinical practice to international relationships*. New York: Jason Aronson.

Yi, K., & Shorter-Gooden, K. (1999). Ethnic identity formation: From stage theory to a constructivist narrative model. *Psychotherapy, 36*(1), 16–26.

Chapter 3
Surviving Together: Individual and Communal Narratives in the Wake of Tragedy

Guiding Questions

What are the forms of trauma that may impact the clients and communities we work with as social workers?

How does narrative theory help us to address the individual and communal impact of trauma?

What do we mean by the term *trauma narrative* and how can it help us understand and assist our clients?

A number of years ago I was attending an interdisciplinary professional conference and was listening to a panel that was addressing a topic that I honestly can't recall. What I do recall is that one of the panelists was talking about trauma and strategies for treating it. A colleague had spotted me from the doorway as she passed by so she came in and sat down next to me to listen. She happens to be a pediatric anesthesiologist. It also happens that English is not her first language. In fact, it's her third. After a moment she leaned over and said, "John, I hear them referring to trauma, but I don't understand. Trauma is like emergency medicine. But what are they talking about?"

As a physician, her immediate association was to the trauma she was all too familiar with in the E.R. She had seen victims of devastating accidents and the aftermath of fires, gunshots, stabbings, and the like, and been part of their medical treatment team. But of course the panel that day was talking about a different kind of trauma—the kind we are addressing in this chapter. Make no mistake, we are still talking about wounds, sometimes quite devastating wounds. But these wounds are psychic and emotional, though there may have been physical ones as well. Some would even say that they are wounds of the soul, and for many of those affected by this kind of trauma, its often hidden impact is felt long after the wounds of the body have healed.

The word trauma actually comes from the Greek word *το τραυμα*, which means *wound*. When we speak of our clients (or ourselves for that matter) who have experienced trauma, we are talking about the wounds that they have sustained in the course of their living. These are wounds to which we are susceptible because we are human. Having said that, we will see in the course of this chapter that there are predisposing factors, many of which are very familiar to us as social workers, which do make it more likely that someone will be impacted by trauma. Like all wounds, they may result from many different sources and take on many different forms. Some may heal rather quickly while others may have a more enduring, even incapacitating, impact.

Throughout this chapter then, we examine what we mean by the word trauma and the numerous ways it may present itself. We consider trauma from both individual and communal perspectives as well as a variety of events that may be considered potentially traumatogenic (trauma inducing). These may be single, repeated, or compounding (multiple different experiences that have an additive effect) events. As part of this discussion, we explore both post-traumatic stress disorder (PTSD) and what is known as complex trauma. We consider traumas that are caused by human action or inaction, as well as by nature itself. Throughout this discussion we consider the nature and importance of meaning making and the impact it has on the experience of trauma. And of course, what holds this all together for our purposes is narrative. This requires us to understand both the nature of trauma narrative and the ways in which narrative is tied to meaning making and ultimately the healing of these deep but often invisible wounds.

Let's begin with a word about what we mean when we use the word trauma and the subjectivity of individual experience. Inasmuch as trauma refers to the kind of wounds that we have already mentioned, the identification and experience of trauma are deeply personal. This has a couple of implications. First, we know that individuals' reactions to what we may think of as potentially traumatogenic events (e.g., motor vehicle accidents, assault of any kind, combat, exposure to terrorist attacks and other forms of violence, natural disasters) may vary.

If you and I are exposed to the same event (for example the terrorist attack on the Bataclan nightclub in Paris in November of 2015), it is possible that I will experience disturbing posttraumatic symptoms following the experience while you will not. That may of course have to do with the specific nature of my experience on the scene, but it may also have to do with factors that are more particular to me. On the other hand, you and I might be exposed to a different kind of event (an earthquake, for example) and you will be more adversely affected than I will be. The key idea is this: the experience of trauma is subjective (Briere & Scott, 2015; Ford, Grasso, Elhai, & Courtois, 2015; van der Kolk, 2014). Though we know that there are predisposing factors that may make us more susceptible to the experience of trauma, and though there certainly are commonalities in the way trauma presents itself, the response of the individual to the potentially traumatogenic event must be honored. In keeping with this, because you and I come from distinct backgrounds, the narrative we form about the supposedly *same* event will be different. It will have similarities, of course—similarities that may result in what we feel to be a strong bond between us (just ask the children and families of Newtown)—but there will be differences. This is a terribly important point because it relates to the respect we have for the person of the client. We must be careful not to impose on the client some external sense of what the "right" reaction to a given event would be or to compare their reaction to that of others. As we discussed in Chap. 1, narrative is about listening, tuning in to the story of client. Narrative is the point of entry into the client's world and a tool to help them heal from the trauma they have experienced, however they have experienced it.

It is also important that we keep in mind that the nature of trauma extends far beyond the boundaries of PTSD (Courtois & Ford, 2013). We will see many men, women, and children who have been adversely affected by traumatic experiences. However, it is likely that only a segment of these individuals will meet the criteria for PTSD. This requires us to be familiar with the nature and manifestations of trauma and to be able to recognize the signs of those wounds when they are present.

Trauma Narrative and Meaning Making

When we speak of trauma narrative we are referring to the story of a traumatic event or series of events and the ways in which these have impacted the life of the teller. As we have been discussing, the narrative impulse (Riessman, 2008) that we all share leads us to recount our experience in the form of a story. But trauma can have a powerful impact on that narrative instinct, and our ability to craft that story. Pierre Janet (1859–1947), one of the earliest theorists to explore the nature of trauma, made a distinction between traumatic memory and narrative memory. For Janet, traumatic memory involved the individual reliving the past experience as though it were present. This might come in the form of flashbacks or other phenomena that kept the person from giving the trauma its proper place in the past. Narrative memory on the other hand allowed the individual to situate the traumatic experience in the context of their history in a way that enabled them to move on (Janet (1925) as cited in Hunt & McHale, 2008). In a similar vein, Shohet (2007) contrasts *stable* and *authentic* narratives. Stable narratives, she suggests, are coherent and provide an orderly account of events and their place in one's history. Authentic narratives, on the other hand, may express a lack of clarity or ambivalence as the individual is struggling to develop an understanding of the event or events in question and their place in the person's overall life experience.

Another way of conceptualizing this is to note that the experience of trauma often results in what is referred to as a broken narrative (Hyden & Brockmeier, 2008; Ladegaard, 2015). These stories may be filled with gaps and inconsistencies some of which have to do with missing information (e.g., the client who doesn't remember or is confused about "what happened next"), a fluctuating emotional and cognitive response to the experience of the trauma expressed as a shifting perspective or attitude about the event, or difficulty locating the trauma in the overall context of their life and sense of self. This may at times be expressed as questions like "How did this happen to me?" or thoughts such as "I'm not the kind of person who …" In these instances, clients are renegotiating their sense of identity and personal history to find a way to accommodate the experience of trauma and discern a path forward. It is in this way, I suggest, that narrative approaches to treatment can be particularly helpful.

This effort to renegotiate a sense of oneself and one's history ties in directly to what I have already suggested is a key consideration in a narrative approach to trauma—the way we make meaning of experience. The issue of whether or not people even attempt to make meaning out of traumatic experiences has been a matter of some debate. Some have reported findings suggesting that following a potentially traumatic event like 9/11, many people did not attempt in any specific way to make meaning of the experience (Rennicke, 2007). However, this has at times been assessed by directly asking individuals affected if they tried (i.e., in a purposeful and conscious way) to make meaning of such events. Others meanwhile have suggested that meaning making is an intrinsic human activity in which we are continually engaged (McTighe & Tosone, 2015). This latter point of view, I suggest, is consistent with the position of this book that human beings are storied creatures who are continually crafting the narrative of our life experience. We do this as part and parcel of our nature and functioning. While in the context of psychotherapy, for example, the effort to make meaning of a traumatic event or events (or any experience for that matter) may be undertaken in a more deliberate way, perhaps at the prompting of a narratively informed or oriented therapist, we human beings are always making meaning of experience. It is important to note, however, that this does not necessarily imply that the meaning we derive will feel pleasant or even necessarily be life-giving or healing.

There are a number of authors who have addressed this predilection for meaning making quite eloquently. Perhaps the most well known of these is Viktor Frankl (1905–1997). Frankl was an Austrian Jewish psychiatrist and neurologist who was imprisoned in several Nazi concentration camps during World War II. His experience of living and witnessing such extraordinary adversity as well as his own and others' responses to it contributed to his development of Logotherapy. Frankl strove to articulate what he saw as the indispensible existential importance of making meaning of suffering in order to access inner resources that could lead to survival and transformation (Frankl, 1946/1984). Frankl wrote,

> We must never forget that we may also find meaning even when confronted with a hopeless situation, when facing a fate that cannot be changed. For what then matters is to bear witness to the uniquely human potential at its best, which is to transform a personal tragedy into a triumph, to turn one's predicament into a human achievement… In some way, suffering ceases to be suffering at the moment it finds a meaning, such as the meaning of sacrifice (p. 135).

Though meaning is of existential importance at all times, it may be most purposefully sought in times of trauma, loss, and suffering. For both individuals and communities, the meaning that is made of adversity can have a significant impact on the psychosocial consequences of it (Fullerton, 2004). Narrative is deeply important here inasmuch as it provides the framework within which we make sense of loss and suffering (Neimeyer, 2005). The challenge of trauma is that it may shatter the established ways in which we have previously understood our self, life, and the world.

This notion is central to the thinking of Janoff-Bulman (1992) whose work is of seminal importance in this area. Janoff-Bulman proposes that human beings have a conceptual set of assumptions about the world and the way it works. These are organized hierarchically so that the most fundamental assumptions are the most basic and least open to change. Janoff-Bulman suggests that there are three such assumptions. The world is benevolent. The world is meaningful. The self is worthy.

Now while the vicissitudes of life may seem to challenge these assertions and the suggestion that they are fundamental to our human perspective, I'd ask you to give them serious consideration. Janoff-Bulman suggests that these conceptual foundations are rooted in the earliest part of our development and are connected to what has been conceived of as a sense of basic trust (Erikson, 1968), a reliable holding environment (Winnicott, 1965), a reasonably secure attachment to a caregiver or caregivers (Bowlby, 1969, 1973), or the fruit of a sufficiently consistent environment through our representation of interactions that have become generalized (RIGS) (Stern, 1985). If we think about it, though life may be far from perfect, most of the time most people get enough of what they need emotionally and psychologically to continue hoping and even believing in life, the world and themselves, at least to a sufficient enough extent that they continue moving forward. Some may find that they agree with Janoff-Bulman's assertions philosophically, even if they struggle with one or more of them on a personal level. In those instances, that philosophical or intellectual belief in the benevolence and meaningfulness of the world, and the worthiness of the self, is what they rely on to continue their journey.

The problem, Janoff-Bulman says, is that when we are subjected to trauma, these assumptions we hold about the world are shattered and with them the meaning that we make of our existence. These shattered assumptions must be renegotiated if we are to reestablish our balance in life, to heal, and to be able to carry on. Some will engage in this process spontaneously and maybe even without conscious reflection and restore enough belief in the world and themselves to reestablish a sense of normalcy in their life. Though they might benefit from some assistance or support with this in the form of therapy, many will not avail themselves of it for one reason or another. Others, however, will do so. They will find their way to people like us (just as we ourselves may seek out the help of another to work through the traumas we experience) and ask for our support as they struggle with life narratives that have been fractured, and as they struggle to regain or even discover for the first time a sense of meaning.

Janoff-Bulman (1992) goes on to suggest that there are three principal strategies by which people reestablish their sense of the benevolence of the world, the meaningfulness of life, and their own goodness. The first of these is comparison. We are likely all familiar with the instinct to compare ourselves and our fate to that of others. How often have you heard someone comment about how, even though they are struggling with their own challenges, they know there are people who have it far worse? Most people derive some degree of comfort from knowing that they are not alone and that others have a greater share of suffering to bear than they do. Secondly, people interpret the role they have to play in the trauma or other suffering they have endured. This itself can take on two forms. For some it becomes a reflection of who they are rather than a statement about the world (e.g., "There must be something wrong with *me*."). For others, coming to an understanding of the part they have played in their own suffering (even apart from the "objective" truth of that assessment) and viewing it perhaps as the result of a strategic error or bad decision on their part can help restore some sense of perceived control (e.g., "If only I hadn't decided to walk home alone so late at night." "Something told me not to go there that day, I should have paid attention!").

When faced with the lack of control that trauma so commonly represents, this effort comes from individuals' desire to restore a sense of their own control and agency. However, as therapists listening to the narratives that are implicit in these efforts, we need to attend to the negative effects that an attitude of self-blame can cause in victims of trauma. It is important to remember that there are many people whose traumas have conditioned them to accept blame for the actions of others even when this is strikingly inaccurate and even more harmful to them.

A young man named Rob with whom I once worked had, prior to my meeting him, moved to a city on the West Coast for a new job he had accepted. Being new to town and knowing no one he was eager to make friends. He had only been there about a month when he readily accepted an invitation from some co-workers to go out for happy hour one Friday after work. Happy hour turned into dinner and settling in with his co-workers for what turned out to be a rather long evening. Returning home to his apartment complex sometime after midnight, Rob drove around the back of his building to where the garages were. Each apartment was assigned a single, separate garage space. He parked his car and as he emerged from the garage several men attacked him. He was never totally certain of their number but he felt sure that there were at least three. They beat him severely, rendering him unconscious.

When he awoke sometime later he was in the back seat of the car on the floor. At least one of the men was seated in the back and he could hear the voices of others in the front. He could feel blood running from the top of his head and from his mouth. He struggled to breathe. He thought he would die. Somehow in the midst of all this he had the presence of mind not to alert the attackers to the fact that he was now conscious. It seemed that they drove for quite a while, though he had no idea where they were, nor how long he had been unconscious.

At some point the car came to a stop. Rob heard the doors open and the men get out. He was then dragged from the back seat of the car by his feet. He was beaten again and was stripped naked by the assailants who got back in the car and left. After they drove away he lay there for some time fearing to move. It was winter and the impact of the cold began to set in as he lay naked on the ground. He knew that he needed to find shelter and help. He struggled to pull himself up and look around. He was by the waterfront in what was largely a warehouse and shipping district. He saw no one around but focused on a lighted window about half a block away.

With a great deal of pain and effort Rob made his way to building with the light in the window. It turned out to be a shipping company that was open throughout the night. He opened the door and entered the office where a woman sat at the desk. It was all he could do to say, "Help me," before he collapsed on the floor. The office worker was of course horrified. She immediately called 911. Rob later told me that in that moment he felt so many things: gratitude for being alive, relief at finding someone to help him, the comforting warmth of the office, embarrassment at lying there naked in front of a strange woman, and both searing pain and terror over what he had just endured.

He was released from the hospital a couple of days later with several broken ribs, a broken nose, and a number of stitches in his head. He was severely bruised and sore. His car had been recovered only a couple of miles from where he was left by the attackers. Police were searching for the perpetrators but had little evidence to work with. It turned out that there had been a couple of other nighttime robberies around his apartment complex. Car windows had been smashed; another car was stolen and not recovered. The detective on his case guessed that he had simply been in the wrong place at the wrong time.

About a week later, Rob attempted to return to work. He hadn't been sleeping, and he had a great deal of difficulty concentrating. He tried to shake off the images and the fear that always came with them. He tried not to look constantly over his shoulder, especially when he was alone, and even more so when he went home. In spite of his efforts, it didn't take long for him to feel that he could no longer handle it. His parents were deeply concerned about him. They had flown out to be with him the morning after the assault, and cared for him for almost a week. They offered to stay longer but Rob insisted that he was fine and that they had their own lives to get back to. In addition, he was going back to work anyway and there would be little point in them hanging around. They continued to call Rob every day to check on him. At first he tried to convince them, and himself, that everything was fine. When he finally admitted that he was in fact not fine at all, they encouraged him to come home. Rob quit his job and moved back to the East Coast. I met him just about a week later.

When Rob first shared with me the story of his trauma, I felt that what he most needed at the moment was safety and support. Having returned to his parents' home, Rob had the benefits of a familiar physical environment where he felt about as safe as anyone might. He had a positive, loving relationship with his parents who were doing their best to help him, though he said that he knew they were "a bit out of their element." Rob had decided not to look for another job quite yet, and his parents were supportive of that. Nonetheless, they were trying to carry on with the semblance of a normal life, chatting about the news and their day, suggesting to Rob that he get out for some exercise or reconnect with his friends. His physical injuries were just about healed and they so very much wished that his internal wounds would be healed as well.

But Rob felt that his life was on pause. He described feeling disoriented, preoccupied, "out of it." His anxiety was elevated. This sometimes came in the form of being easily startled or feeling nervous for no apparent reason. He had difficulty sleeping, even with some medicine his physician had prescribed. Occasionally he experienced intrusive memories of the attack, and with these at times a subtle detail would return, unexplained. One day he told me that he had remembered the smell of the carpet on the floor of the car and the feeling of the dirt or grit that had inevitably been carried in on people's shoes.

But most of all, Rob struggled with trying to make sense of it all—all that had happened to him and the consequences of it. There was the assault and the fear that he would be killed, of course. But there was more. There was the excitement he had experienced about his new job, the adventure of the move to a new city. Rob told me he was always a confident person, ready to take on new challenges. There were the fantasies and wishes he had for his future—professionally and personally. But now it felt like that was all gone and his view of the future was foggy at best and empty at worst. This fear and uncertainty were deeply unfamiliar to him. He felt like he had lost himself. And therein lay our most important work.

I could provide Rob with all kinds of psychoeducation about trauma and its sequelae. I could normalize so many aspects of what he was experiencing; and all of that was helpful. But mostly what Rob and I did was work on renegotiating his sense of self. It is important to note here that I do not say "restoring" his sense of self. After what Rob had lived through, there was no question of simply going back to the way things were, even the way he understood and related to himself and others. There would be continuity in his sense of self; but things would inevitably be different. Rob's narrative of himself, the world, and himself *in* the world was being re-crafted. He was struggling to come to a new sense of meaning and heal, as Janoff-Bulman might suggest, the assumptions about life that had been shattered.

As might be expected, Rob's narrative about this traumatic turn in his story evolved and took a number of twists and turns. At times there was a tone of bitterness and fear as he told the story of how awful and untrustworthy people were and what a harsh place the world was. At other times, he did indeed blame himself. "What was I thinking staying out so late? I should have been more attentive when I drove around to those garages. I should have known better. Why didn't I fight back? Maybe I could have scared them away ..." At still other times, he was enraged, fantasizing about what he would do to the perpetrators if he could find them, and unbearably frustrated that he could not.

As we worked together over a period of some months Rob did begin to experience greater peace and integration. His acute symptoms subsided as we began to establish a new story, a new sense of meaning. I had not had the benefit of knowing Rob prior to his enduring this trauma, so I asked him to tell me about himself in some detail—not just the facts and figures, so to speak, but the story of him as a person. I wanted to know the story of Rob, what he was like before his trauma. As he told me that story, we were able to connect more and more to the ways in which that Rob was still present. As the fog began to clear, Rob discovered so many points of continuity between his sense of himself at that time and prior to the assault. He still enjoyed the same things, and felt the same way about the important people in his life. And particularly when his anger was not overtaking him, he knew that he still held the same core values he always had.

Nonetheless, Rob knew that he was different. He had been changed by what he had endured. At first he felt defeated by this realization; he had hoped that he would just go back to being his "old self"—something his parents and others suggested to him at times in the most well-intentioned way. I, however, strove to reassure Rob that such a change was expectable. Though no one could predict exactly how the change would manifest itself over time, I would say, how could one go back to a time when such a traumatic experience had not happened? Of course he would be different. But the remainder of the story, the future, was his to craft.

Eventually, Rob noticed that while he was different, he was also still himself. He experienced comfort in recognizing that continuity, but was also clear that he felt he had become more "serious" as he would put it. He felt a greater sense of guardedness even though he had begun to open himself to new experiences. He had started doing things with friends and was looking for a job. Though there were still moments when he felt angry over what had happened to him and could even get somewhat lost in those thoughts if he indulged them, he also had a great sense of gratitude and was keenly aware of the aspects of his life that were most meaningful to him and in which he felt the most promise for his future.

Let's return to the work of Janoff-Bulman (1992). The third strategy she highlights for restoring our positive assumptions about the world is the search for benefit in the trauma or a sense of the purpose for which this might have happened. In the wake of even a terribly painful experience, this approach can help traumatized individuals regain a sense of the orderliness and meaningfulness of the world and of experience. Though it may not be the first place our mind goes when we think of trauma, it is nonetheless important to highlight that the outcome of trauma and its impact on our narrative are not universally negative. In fact, there is abundant research that has highlighted the way in which people have found growth and even benefit in the wake of trauma.

Affleck and Tennen (1996), for example, discuss the importance of benefit-finding and benefit-reminding. As they attempt to cope with traumatic or other adverse circumstances, people will search for benefits that have been gained or remind themselves of positive aspects of the life situation in which they find themselves. Associated with improved coping and reduced levels of distress, these strategies include a strengthening of relationships, positive changes to the personality, and a turn to deeper values, priorities, and goals. Additionally, individuals who find benefit in their circumstances may experience reduced feelings of victimization and a greater sense of mastery and meaning.

What is unclear, Affleck and Tennen note, is whether the benefit-finding and benefit-reminding lead to enhanced coping or whether, in fact, it is the other way around. Perhaps those who are better adjusted are able to find some benefit in their situation. In other words, is the ability to find benefit even in the wake of a traumatic event a dispositional trait, a feature of the personality that leads to improved coping, or is it an approach that may be undertaken purposefully in order to enhance coping? This is certainly a question that requires additional research. From a clinical point of view, I suggest that with proper pace and timing, listening for, highlighting, and even encouraging expressions of benefit in the evolving narrative of our clients is a positive strategy to enhance coping. At the same time, however, we must acknowledge that some individuals will have an easier time with this than others, and we must proceed gently and patiently.

Elsewhere in the literature the dynamic associated with benefit finding is referred to as posttraumatic growth (PTG) (Calhoun & Tedeschi, 2006a, 2006b; Janoff-Bulman, 2006; Tedeschi & Calhoun, 1995, 2004). Calhoun and Tedeschi (2006a), for example, suggest that growth may happen in several different ways. Individuals may experience growth following trauma as a change in the way they view themselves, the way they relate to others, or even their overall philosophy of life.

A related vein of research has considered the distinction between meaning making as making sense of a traumatic event and meaning making as benefit finding (Davis & Nolen-Hoeksema, 2001; Davis, Nolen-Hoeksema, & Larson, 1998; Davis, Wortman, Lehman, & Silver, 2000). In other words, while it is possible for people to emerge from a traumatic experience having discovered benefits that have enhanced their life in some way, it is also possible more simply to find an explanation that fits into a person's worldview. However, that explanation is not necessarily positive. For example, in a study of social workers' effort to make meaning personally and professionally of the events of 9/11, results showed that some participants arrived at a meaning that had a negative emotional valence (McTighe & Tosone, 2015).

The shift that Rob experienced in his narrative offers us the opportunity to consider the work of some other scholars who have addressed this process following trauma. Park and Folkman (1997) propose a broad distinction between what they refer to as global and situational meaning. In a tone that is reminiscent of the work of Janoff-Bulman (1992), Park and Folkman suggest that global meaning is the broadest level of our assumptions and beliefs about ourselves and the world in which we live. Situational meaning involves the way in which we make sense of the specific circumstances in which we may find ourselves at any particular time. Global and situational meanings have an interdependent, recursive relationship in that each informs and challenges the other. Park and Folkman's work is quite nuanced and merits a consideration beyond the scope of what we can cover here.

For our purposes, I would highlight their position that when we are faced with adversity such as trauma we enter into a process through which we seek to accommodate that traumatic experience into our sense of life and the world. Not surprisingly, this most often happens by trying to fit the particular situation in which we find ourselves or the event we have endured into our overall framework of meaning—our global meaning. If our sense of global meaning is challenged beyond what it can bear and thus is not able to contain the present situation, then that global framework itself much change to accommodate the new experience. This is, as you might image, much more challenging inasmuch as it represents a shift in the fundamental story of our selves, the world, and our selves in the world.

Returning for a moment to the story of Rob, we can see this process in action. Through the trauma he endured, Rob's global narrative was fractured in a way that left him feeling shaken and confused. He struggled not only to make sense of the assault itself, but also how he was to move on in his life. His world no longer seemed to make sense, nor did he know quite where and how he fit in it. Ultimately, his sense of himself and his identity as "continuous but nonetheless changed" and his sense of the world as a different place than he had previously experienced (but one that he was learning how to negotiate) represented a shift in his global framework or narrative of meaning—one that allowed him to come to a reasonable accommodation of the trauma he endured and find a way forward.

This perspective is also consistent with Neimeyer's (2001a, 2001b, 2005, 2006) understanding of the way in which the coherence of our narratives of self and the world are challenged by the experience of loss. Just as Park and Folkman (1997) refer to global and situational meaning, Neimeyer (2004) refers to the way in which the *micro-narratives* of our day-to-day experience fit into and at times challenge the *macro-narrative* that provides our understanding of the world and shapes how we interact with and respond to it. Once again, when that narrative framework is shaken, we are left confused and uncertain about what sense to make of our self and our life. This takes us back to the kind of renegotiation process that we have been discussing so far.

The Varieties of Trauma and Its Manifestations

At this point let us examine some of the ways in which trauma may occur as well as the varied manifestations of its impact in our lives. A comprehensive review of what is known about trauma falls well outside the scope of this chapter and this book. There are any number of excellent sources that you might consult if you'd like to understand trauma more fully from biological, psychological, social, and even spiritual perspectives. Similarly, a wonderful breadth of material is available to you representing a wide variety of perspectives to deepen your clinical skills. For our purposes, we will stay focused on a narrative understanding of and approach to trauma.

To begin, we may consider the distinction that was mentioned earlier in the chapter between post-traumatic stress disorder (PTSD) and other forms of trauma including what we refer to as complex trauma (Courtois & Ford, 2013). It is worth noting that in the current fifth edition of the Diagnostic and Statistical Manual of Mental Disorders (DSM-5) (American Psychiatric Association, 2013), PTSD was taken out of the Anxiety Disorders section and has now been given its own chapter, Trauma- and Stressor-Related Disorders. This accomplishes a couple of things. While survivors of trauma do commonly experience anxiety and other anxiety-based reactions, the creation of a separate chapter in DSM-5 acknowledges trauma as a clinical phenomenon of its own, with varied manifestations and sequelae, as well as the multiple areas of life that may be affected by it (Briere & Scott, 2015). Secondly, the new criteria capture more broadly both dissociative symptoms and the persistent impact of trauma on one's sense of self and engagement with life. This offers greater room for the recognition of complex trauma and complex posttraumatic stress.

If you are like most people, you are probably more familiar with the notion of, or at least the term, PTSD than any other particularly nuanced expression of trauma. The phrase PTSD has found its way into the lexicon of nonspecialists when discussing the impact of potentially traumatic events, and has even become a part of fairly ordinary speech. Without going into all of its diagnostic criteria, PTSD refers to the adverse impact of "exposure to actual or threatened death, serious injury, or sexual violence" (American Psychiatric Association, 2013, p. 271) on psychological, biological, and social functioning. We think, for example, of soldiers in combat zones or law enforcement professionals, the victims of natural disasters such as floods and earthquakes, and those affected by terrorist attacks. Other examples include the victims of severe motor vehicle accidents, robberies, fires, and physical and sexual assault. We think of individuals (who often enough identify themselves with a group or class of people like themselves) who were exposed to an event or events that radically disrupted their sense of self and the way they see and interact with the world.

A student of mine once shared with me that he had formerly been a New York City Firefighter. He was a chauffeur—a fire truck driver—and he drove one of the first fire trucks to respond into the plaza of the Twin Towers on the morning of 9/11. Though we talked about this a number of years after the event, he described his experience to me in some graphic detail that does not bear repeating here. He was only in his 40s, but was retired with disability. With a dose of dark humor, he told me about seeing his former colleagues periodically when they went for checkups at clinics that had been organized for them. They would go from one area to the next having all aspects of their health assessed. The last station, he told me, was always psychiatry. Afterwards, he said, they would all stand around on the street outside, many of them smoking (an irony that was not lost on him). As each one emerged in turn, they would ask,

> "So what about you? You got PTSD?"
> "Oh yeah," would come the reply, "I got PTSD. What about you?"
> "Yeah, me too ... See you next time!"

Though they would speak of it in this superficially lighthearted way as a function of their coping, my student knew that his friends were still impacted just as he was by intrusive thoughts and flashbacks, feelings of avoidance, hyperarousal, and all the rest—an experience that they continued to struggle with day to day. Regardless of how one has come to have PTSD, the symptoms can be devastatingly impactful. They can dominate the daily living of the person affected, taking over their narratives and meaning making, and making life before the trauma seem elusive.

While there is similarity between PTSD and what is referred to as complex trauma or complex posttraumatic stress, there are also important differences that must be noted—differences that have a direct effect on the narratives of its victims. Complex trauma refers to "severe, prolonged, and repeated trauma, almost always of an interpersonal nature, often beginning early in life" (Briere & Scott, 2015, p. 54). This sort of trauma is born not of a single event, but of the cumulative impact of psychological and physical injury sustained over time. It is the kind of wound that commonly has a severe impact not only on the developing sense of self of the victim, but together with that, on their ability to manage interpersonal boundaries, relate to others, and regulate their affect.

In order to handle the sometimes seismic shifts in their perception of themselves and the world, they may learn to rely on dissociation or any one of a number of tension reduction strategies that often enough can lead to further difficulties in their own right. These may include things like risk-taking behaviors (indiscriminant sex, driving at high speeds, frequenting places known to be dangerous), cutting and other forms of self-harm, suicidal gestures, eating-disordered behaviors, and substance use (Briere & Scott, 2015). From a treatment point of view, it is of the utmost importance not to get so caught up in these self-regulatory behaviors that we lose sight of or fail to see the trauma that is their origin.

Understood narratively, while we need to attend to these problematic tension reduction strategies as they present themselves in treatment, we must continue to listen for the story of the wound(s) that gives rise to them. In fact, as a means of perceived self-preservation, our traumatized clients might even attempt, consciously or unconsciously, to occupy our attention with these more acute behaviors and concerns as a way of keeping us both—therapist *and* client—from opening and exploring the Pandora's Box of traumas of which they are often so terrified.

Of course, it is essential that we attend to behaviors like suicidality, cutting, and risk taking that put our clients in harm's way, but when we are talking about trauma, I encourage you to hear these things in the context of the larger story of their woundedness, to hold them carefully and patiently and not lose sight of the work of healing that remains. Whether your client has PTSD or has been subjected to cumulative trauma their whole life, that kind of patient attention is essential. To view any such client in a reductionistic way that attended to the troubling and even frustrating nature of their behaviors without holding their trauma in the forefront of our minds would do them a great disservice. We will talk more about this stance of patience and other issues that bear on treatment shortly. For now, let's look further at the manifestations of trauma.

Having explored the distinction between PTSD and complex trauma, we can consider trauma from a different point of view: individual vs. communal trauma. In some sense, all trauma is individual. Trauma happens to individual people, whether singly or in groups. Posttraumatic reactions, even in the wake of large-scale events, are experienced by and vary among individuals. But there is more to the story here. When we think of potentially traumatogenic events from an individual point of view, our attention is drawn to things like motor vehicle and other accidents, sexual or physical assault, interpersonal or other forms of violence, and witnessing of a horrific event that happens to another person.

Some of these individual traumas may occur once at any point in the life cycle or they may be endured over an extended period of time, perhaps beginning in childhood. The traumatic impact of the event may be immediate and readily apparent, or it may linger in the background, hidden sometimes even to its victim, showing itself in subtle ways that may not readily seem connected to the trauma. I have found myself on numerous occasions assessing a new client who has come to me to work on an issue that feels immediate and pressing, but the origins of which they see as more elusive. "I have no idea why I started doing that, feeling that way ...." A thorough history taking sometimes reveals a potential trauma in their past (or sometimes even in their present) that when explored reveals itself as the source of their current distress in a way that may feel astounding to the client.

This is for me an example of one of the more compelling dimensions of narrative practice. A narrative approach to treatment is not about being an audience for a scripted and rehearsed story that the client has to tell you. In fact, when you sense that the story has been scripted and rehearsed I suggest that there is likely a deeper story that underlies it, and a whole lot more to be discovered. Knowing that oftentimes there are aspects of our *own* stories that are not readily apparent to us, narrative practice is about helping the client to explore and even uncover the story that is there to be told and that, in being told, holds the promise of growth, healing, and discovery of new ways of living.

A particular class of these traumas is found among combat veterans so many of whom have experienced unspeakable horrors—horrors that may overwhelmingly alter their narratives and which they may have an extraordinarily hard time putting into words. The present generation of soldiers, sailors, and airmen who have returned and continue to return from combat in Iraq and Afghanistan are demonstrating noteworthy levels of mental health difficulties including posttraumatic stress (Ramchand, Rudavsky, Grant, Tanielian, & Joycox, 2015). At present, an average of 20 of these veterans are committing suicide on a daily basis (Shane & Kime, 2016). Additionally, a relationship has been demonstrated between deployment to Iraq and Afghanistan and aggressive and violent behavior among members of the military (MacManus et al., 2015). The trauma that they have endured has produced psychological and physiological changes in them, even at times altering their very perception of violence, a phenomenon sometimes referred to as combat addiction (Hecker, Hermenau, Crombach, & Elbert, 2015). It is a change that is being addressed and likely requires even more attention and resources.

For those who have survived natural and man-made disasters, the individual and communal impact of trauma can similarly be intense and enduring. The victims of an event like Hurricane Katrina and the earthquakes in 2010 in Haiti or in the summer of 2016 in Rome, and those caught in the path of wildfires and floodwaters, are left to deal not only with the experience of the event itself, but also with its environmental and personal aftermath stretching on weeks, months, and even years. Survivors of man-made events like the Holocaust, 9/11, Newtown, Las Vegas and other instances of mass shootings grapple with the impact of loss that touches them as individuals, families, and communities. In the case of Holocaust survivors, the sheer enormity of the horror has resulted in a multigenerational legacy that has shaped the lives of the children and now grandchildren of its survivors (Yehuda et al., 2016). These kinds of multi-victim events are both public and personal (Aldrich & Kallivayalil, 2016) and so they shape the stories not only of individuals, but also of the communities that they touch. As we discussed in chapter one, individual narratives shape the communal narrative which recursively shapes the individual. Following 9/11, attention was drawn to the public and communal nature of our mourning, a shared grief that has been written about and ritualized ever since (Kitch, 2003).

The narratives that flow from such large-scale events relate not only the story of individual and collective losses, but also our efforts to make sense of them. They reveal an evolving social dialogue about fear, loss, outrage, and our response to them. These narratives come in the form of political speeches, policy initiatives, and op-eds. There are hero stories that hold up the best of who we are (e.g., narratives of first responders and their often unimaginable bravery, stories of those who go beyond themselves to serve their community in times of such great need). And there are efforts on the part of special interest groups from across the ideological spectrum to position themselves in the face of tragedy to support and even advance the beliefs of their constituents. The gun-control debates that flare up in the wake of events like the mass shooting at the Pulse nightclub in Orlando in the spring of 2016, or in Las Vegas in October of 2017 are seen by some as an effort to politicize a tragedy, and by others as the final straw that must finally result in the realization that the place of guns in American culture has to change. In the midst of all of this, I encourage you to hear an evolving communal narrative—in this case a narrative of trauma that touches us all directly or indirectly. In the years since 9/11, the narrative that Americans tell themselves about their sense of relative safety in the world has been altered inexorably, changing not only how we travel, but also how we look at each other and the world.

Narrative Approaches to the Treatment of Trauma

At this point let us turn our attention to some issues related to narrative approaches to trauma treatment. Note that I refer here to *approaches*—in the plural. That is because, while they may share some epistemological foundations and even bear some resemblance to each other, narrative forms of treatment do not, in my view, represent a cookie cutter way of working with clients and their stories. This applies

When a loss is even more public, affecting not only an individual or a family, but a community, the effect can be even further magnified. Consider the situation for those impacted by an event such as a homicide (Aldrich & Kallivayalil, 2016). In this case, individuals and communities are challenged not only by the difficulty of tolerating the pain of another, but also frankly by the inclination to lose interest. Think, for example, of tragedies that happen on a fairly public stage (e.g., mass shootings at schools or public venues). Media coverage is intense. There is widespread interest and concern, particularly for those whose lives have been lost. Their stories are told; vigils are held. There is a public outpouring of support. But when the television crews leave the scene and the news cycle moves on, when schools and shops and nightclubs reopen, and life goes back to a perhaps *new* normal, there is grief that remains and narratives that continue to evolve—removed from the public's eyes.

Still another example is found in survivors of suicide—parents, spouses, children, friends, and other loved ones. For so many, the pressure to move on and heal is compounded by the perception of shame and even scandal that for so many still surrounds suicide. At events to promote awareness of suicide (see organizations such as the American Foundation for Suicide Prevention at www.afsp.org, for example), the power of survivors who gather with photos of lost loved ones to share the stories of *their* lives and pain, and the grief that binds them together, is remarkable. There is, in a sense, a joining of narratives. Survivors become the living witnesses of the struggles of those they have lost even as they live with the narrative of their own loss and survivorship. Those who gather together at each event craft a shared narrative that speaks to the common bond of the pain they share. Speaking out about this, engaging in activism, and finding a common bond—these strategies are often experienced as deeply helpful. But for so many others, this story remains untold.

Case Example

A woman named Catherine once presented for treatment due to the return of a depression that she had been struggling with on and off for about 10 years. In her early 60s, Catherine was attractive, and well dressed. Her hair and makeup were done with careful attention. She was soft spoken and articulate. Her symptom profile led easily to a diagnosis of a recurrent major depressive disorder. Less clear were the origins of her illness. She had no history of depression prior to the point in time, 10 years earlier, when she experienced her first symptoms. There was no family history of depression, and no apparent genetic predisposition. Her symptoms commonly began in the late summer or early fall and usually dissipated sometime in the beginning of winter. Throughout the months in between, she had a difficult time functioning. Catherine was a housewife. Her children were grown; only one was still at home. Her husband went to work every morning and returned in the evening. When depressed, she could spend the entire day in bed, sometimes tearful, sometimes feeling that there were no tears left to be shed. And she had no clear idea why.

ing their therapist as they come to session and tell the same or a similar story every week. In these cases, they are likely projecting onto the clinician what they have heard or experienced from others. It can be challenging for these clients to imagine that we might be there with them willingly and patiently, and with genuine and sustained interest and concern.

Even though we might experience this phenomenon with any number of clients, it may be especially true for those who have experienced a trauma that others, whether in their immediate circle or even the public at large, are aware of. In these instances, supportive people may be so invested in the return to normalcy and the wish that those affected by trauma feel "better" that they push those involved to move on from their feelings. I have seen this happen with clients who have been the victims of armed robbery, for example. They are told that they have to go on with their life and that they mustn't be controlled by fear. This is likely well intentioned of course. Think about how difficult it is to see someone you love living in fear or pain. But it is a far easier thing to say than do. Sometimes, it leads traumatized individuals to simply stop sharing their pain.

A woman was once brought into an agency where I worked by a friend of hers. She didn't have an appointment, but she was visibly distraught—sobbing and not able to talk about what was upsetting her. Since I happened to be available, the receptionist called and asked if I could come out to help. I sat the two women down in a nearby office to try to understand what was going on. The friend told me that the woman's daughter had died. I expressed support and concern and focused on helping the woman feel calmer in the moment. Meanwhile, the friend, trying to be supportive was saying, "You have to calm down. You have to stop this. It isn't healthy. Your daughter will never rest in peace if you keep this up!" Though I was somewhat taken aback, I could tell she meant well. Nonetheless, I gently but firmly stopped her. I asked the woman *when* her daughter had died. "Four days ago," she said. She had just been buried the day before! I reassured her that her reaction was quite "normal" and offered ongoing support. Again, her friend truly was trying to be helpful. From a narrative perspective, however, we might reflect on how difficult it is to sit with the pain of another person, particularly a loved one. This can be something we lose sight of in the context of our own self-narrative about who we are and what we do as social workers. It also speaks to the underlying social and cultural narrative about grief and what it *should* look like. In this case, her friend's grief led this woman to bring her to a mental health clinic the day after her daughter's burial, believing that her suffering was cause for concern.

In perhaps an even more powerful way, there are social groups who share a narrative that reinforces the notion that no one on the "outside" will understand the story, experiences, and feelings they share. This is extraordinarily common, for example, among veterans, members of law enforcement, and other first responders—groups that are commonly inclined only to share with one of their own. You may have already tuned into how challenging the private nature of this narrative can be, given the prevalence of trauma in these communities. For this reason, groups that facilitate this kind of sharing (e.g., hotlines that allow vets to talk to other vets who are trained to listen and help, programs that encourage and sometimes even require members to access needed services) are so important.

she could. Since she had a hard time expressing herself, I suggested that she imagine a big red button on the corner of my desk—a stop button. If at any point she felt that things were too upsetting she could simply hit that button and we would stop what we were talking about. She nodded her agreement. Sure enough we arrived after a few minutes at questions about her childhood; she paused and hit the imaginary red button on the corner of my desk. She looked over at me to see my reaction. Without questioning her, I said, "Ok. Let's stop." I sat back in my chair. She smiled and we moved on another topic. Eventually, we did get back to where we left off.

The goal of that strategy of openness is to signal to the client that we are there to work together, to partner with them sensitively—not to force them to go where they are not ready to go. When we work with traumatized individuals (and all clients), it is important to consider that we are not only attending to the story that they tell with their words, but with their bodies as well. We do our best to stay attuned to body language, facial expression, and tone of voice since these will sometimes communicate as much about what clients are experiencing as their words, and sometimes even more.

I have been approaching the story of this work from the angle of the client who fears opening up to discuss their trauma. In this case an image like the therapeutic window helps us decide how much we can encourage the client to delve into their trauma. But it is also important to consider the opposite situation. Sometimes we have clients who have little ability to regulate their own exposure to their trauma or how overwhelmed they get by that exposure. These clients may seem terribly eager to discuss their trauma story, even in detail, even right from the beginning. Especially when we are new to clinical work, we might feel excited to have a client who is so trusting and so willing to work with us. We might even feel gratified that we are getting into this deep material so easily, perhaps congratulating ourselves on how far we have gotten so quickly. However, this is equally a time for caution.

Just as an avoidance of the trauma story can impede therapeutic progress, rapid overexposure can likewise be deeply untherapeutic. These clients can easily get overwhelmed and shut down or decompensate in the face of a flood of memories and emotions (Briere, 2002). It is time to put the brakes on—gently. Reassure your client that you understand how important it is to tell the story, and that you are prepared to hear it all. We don't want the client to fear that they will frighten *us* with their narrative. But let the client know that pacing is important and that you don't want them to get overwhelmed as they explore their narrative. While this can cause some frustration for the client in the moment, it is also a signal that you want the therapeutic space to be safe, and that you will be diligent about maintaining that with and for them. Keep in mind the therapeutic window.

Consistent with what we have said about narrative practice, we will not presume where the client is coming from, what they have experienced, or what their intentions are. We will listen, remain open, and wonder. When working with trauma, as with other kinds of clinical presentations, the stories of our clients and the narrative layers we will uncover together are unique. As we have seen, some may struggle to open up that story to us and even to themselves. Others may have little control over it. Still others may have learned to stop telling the story, even though they need and want to. It is not uncommon to have clients who imagine they are boring or frustrat-

to trauma as much as any other clinical issue. So here I offer you some thoughts, some guidelines about how you might think of and engage in trauma work from a narrative point of view.

When we work with clients who have experienced trauma, in my experience, they often long deeply for a connection that is safe and secure, for the kind of understanding that can bring some relief to the pain they live with as a result of their trauma. But mixed in with that desire is also a great deal of fear—fear of being hurt again, fear of exposure, fear of putting into words the seemingly unspeakable or even of having it uttered aloud by another, and fear of there just not being any words that will do to bear the meaning of what they hold within. In the face of that fear what we must bring are consistency and patience. It has been my experience that clients who are deeply traumatized have told me—maybe even without words—what they need from me. Most commonly, they need me to be still, to be present, and to listen as best I can (Newman, Briere, & Kirlic, 2012). They need me to be open and to wait for them.

So pacing is a terribly important consideration in a narrative approach as it is in all trauma work. Briere and Scott (2015) offer an excellent suggestion for tracking this using the image of the therapeutic window. The authors suggest that there is an important balance to be struck in trauma work between avoidance of the trauma and inundating the client with exposure to the trauma, both of which would be untherapeutic. This balancing point is what he refers to as the therapeutic window. When we work within this therapeutic window, we are encouraging enough exposure to the trauma narrative that the client is able to develop their ability to process it, but not so much exposure that we overwhelm the client's ability to cope or that their self-protective defenses cause them to shut down.

In my experience, when we ask clients to venture with us into waters they perceive to be fraught with danger, it is helpful to offer a sense of our intention. How deep are we going? What if I get scared? I have given an explicit description of the therapeutic window to clients, and this has been at times quite helpful. It has communicated to them the importance of getting into territory that is uncomfortable and even painful and frightening. But it has also provided the reassurance that it is not my intention that they should be overwhelmed. Additionally, it is important to let clients know that they remain in control, something that is often therapeutic in and of itself to traumatized individuals who so commonly feel out of control.

I once saw a woman who was profoundly traumatized and experienced significant dissociative symptoms. Though she was coming for help, she was frightened by even what might seem like the most benign questions on the intake form (e.g., questions about where she grew up, went to school, medical history), wondering why I was asking her about such things. She had a difficult time talking at all. I knew I needed to complete the assessment, but was aware of how frightened she was. I was also aware that I did not know anything about the extent of her trauma and what might be a trigger for her. I decided to show her the intake forms themselves. I let her hold them, flip through them, and read the questions on the pages. I explained that they were routine questions that were asked of everyone who came to the agency for a first appointment. I told her that she didn't have to answer any question that was too upsetting for her. I would ask them one by one, and she would tell me whatever

Case Example

At this point, I'd like you to tune in to what you are thinking and feeling. What are your questions about this case? Hypotheses? What would you explore next?

Consider this. It was late fall when I met Catherine and the weather had turned quite cold. She wore a high turtleneck that rose almost to her jawline, a thick, cable-knit sweater that looked soft and warm. Around her neck, about halfway between her face and shoulders, she wore a gold chain. It was a sturdy chain, but it seemed nonetheless that it had taken some purposeful effort to fasten it over the thickness of the sweater, especially given that it did not fall naturally around the base of her neck, but was suspended from the middle of her collar. A charm dangled from the chain. I could see from a distance that there was an image on the charm, but I couldn't make out clearly what it was.

> "Tell me about your chain, Catherine."
> "Oh," she said, her fingers drawn to it nervously. "That's my Andrew."
> "Who is Andrew?"
> "He was ... *is* my son."

Andrew had struggled through his teen years—problems with friends, problems fitting in. He felt as if he were constantly floundering. There was some drinking and marijuana, and a modest performance in college that didn't yield the sense of direction and purpose they had all hoped for. Was there an undiagnosed depression? His parents had suggested therapy; Andrew resisted. One day in mid-November, 10 years before I met Catherine, she went to Andrew's room with a pile of clean laundry in hand and found him hanging in his closet, dead. She screamed for her husband. Andrew's sister called 911. In the days and weeks after, the whole family was of course devastated and the outpouring of support was impressively generous and deeply helpful. After that jolting pause brought on by the suddenness of their grief, slowly life seemed to begin gathering speed again. Things were getting back to normal—a new normal.

One afternoon a couple of weeks after Andrew's burial, while she was out running errands, Catherine passed by a jewelry store with a display in the window that stopped her in her tracks. It seemed the jeweler could take a photograph of a person and emblazon the image onto a flat metal surface—a plate, a keychain, a charm. Catherine went home and removed Andrew's most recent picture from a frame in the living room. A few days later, she picked up the gold charm with his beautiful face somehow magically preserved right on it. She selected a gold chain, delicate but sturdy. Catherine had worn that chain, and that charm around her neck every day for the past 10 years. Every year, as summer drew to a close and she felt the first cooling of the air, Catherine became depressed: a depression that did not lift until the winter was safely upon her.

In all the years that had passed since Andrew's tragic death, she had never made the connection between the anniversary of his suicide and the depression she experienced every fall. Nor had any of her family. The weight of Andrew's memory around her neck every day was never discussed, never acknowledged, nor was the startling parallel between Catherine's lovely jewelry and the gruesome means by which Andrew had taken his own life. As I tentatively began to explore Catherine's depression as an anniversary reaction, she could not have seemed more puzzled.

"Do you mean to say that ...?"
"How do *you* feel about that, Catherine?" (*wondering with the client* ...).

The narrative that Catherine began to piece together, one she had never even thematized in her own mind and heart, let alone articulated, was of herself as more than a grieving mother. She was a mother who should have known—should have been there—should have walked into that room even minutes earlier. She was a mother who would remain faithful, would never forget, never let go, and never move on as if Andrew were merely a memory.

Catherine and I spent a good deal of time with her story of faithfulness. Having dominated her consciousness for so many years, her narrative was entrenched, unrelenting, and unquestioned. I tried to remain supportive, but not push Catherine in any particular direction. Plenty of people in her life have simply told her to "stop this" and to "move on"—a usually well-intentioned strategy that is rarely successful. It was important to respect the deeply meaningful nature of her story about Andrew's death, her own response of grief, and the witness she bore daily to his memory. It was important to address the impact of finding his body in his room that day, and the effort she has made over the intervening years to keep those images at bay. At the same time, I gently tried to shift some of her attention to her own depression and the toll it took on her life. I tried to listen for what was *not* being said, potential aspects of the story that were missing. We talked together about what it means to grieve and she told me stories of other mothers she knew who had lost children. We talked about the many ways of remembering those we love who have died. A religious woman, we talked about her prayers for Andrew and increasingly for herself, and her conviction that God understood Andrew's pain, and that Andrew was with Him.

Catherine told me that in all the years since Andrew's death she had never talked about him as much as she had during our sessions. She had never spoken of what she had seen that day and how those sights and the raw feelings that accompanied them had lingered in her thoughts and in her dreams. It seemed so important for people to move on, and though Andrew's photos remained in sight, and the crucifix that was used at his funeral hung on the wall in their home, family members, she thought, were reluctant to talk about him for fear of causing her more pain. In point of fact, as she told the story to an attentive witness and we explored it together, her depression began to lighten a bit. Happier memories of Andrew resurfaced in what had been a monolithic story of sadness. There seemed to be more room for the present, for what else was happening in life. The story began to evolve from the unthinkable prospect of leaving Andrew and his memory behind to discovering his uniquely bittersweet and incomparably cherished place in her narrative—a narrative that would in fact go on.

Questions and Activities for Discussion and Further Reflection

Note: The importance of self-care may be particularly worth highlighting in the classroom when discussing trauma. Two concerns should be highlighted. Social workers can be adversely affected by exposure to clients' traumas especially over time. We will discuss this in Chap. 8. Additionally, we must be aware that we may come to this discussion with our own history of trauma, and we need to be attentive to our own triggers and our well-being. This is both for our own benefit and to make sure that our client receives the best care possible.

1. Reflect on your own sense of meaning and meaning making. What are the greatest sources of meaning in your own life? How do these support you, particularly in times of distress or adversity? Do you have a sense of how you have come to this sense of meaning in your life?
2. Janoff-Bulman writes about three fundamental assumptions we carry about the world: The world is benevolent. The world is meaningful. The self is worthy. How do these stack up with your own conscious beliefs and sense of the world? Is this how you see things? Do you struggle with any of these?
3. Have you had the experience of listening to the story of another person's trauma? What is it like for you to sit with that? If you haven't had the experience personally, what do you imagine it will be like? Do you have any concerns or anxieties of your own about being there with them?
4. Search for news items about traumatic events that have affected communities or the wider society. Select items from different sources about the same event. What story do you find them telling about the event? How are they attempting to make meaning of the event? Are there commonalities and/or differences across sources?
5. Did any of the clinical vignettes in the chapter stand out to you or impact you in particular? Which? Reflect on what about that story made an impression on you? Share that with a classmate.
6. Take the case example of Catherine or one of the other clinical examples from the chapter and role-play it in class. Listen for the client's narrative as it emerges and reflect back what you are hearing. Listen for meaning making. Encourage the client in their storytelling but don't rush them.
7. Did reading this chapter make you think of any other kind of trauma that was not explored? Conduct a literature search using terms for that kind of trauma along with the term *narrative*. What do you find? Read one of those articles and share it with classmates as a way of furthering your learning.
8. Articulate for yourself what you understand to be the most important factors in a narrative approach to clinical practice with trauma. Consider how these will impact your presence with your clients.

References

Affleck, G., & Tennen, H. (1996). Construing benefits from adversity: Adaptational significance and dispositional underpinnings. *Journal of Personality, 64*(4), 899–922.

Aldrich, H., & Kallivayalil, D. (2016). Traumatic grief after homicide: Intersections of individual and community loss. *Illness, Crisis, & Loss, 24*(1), 15–33. https://doi.org/10.1177/1054137315587630

American Psychiatric Association. (2013). *Diagnostic and statistical manual of mental disorders* (5th ed.). Washington, DC: American Psychiatric Association.

Bowlby, J. (1969). *Attachment and loss, Vol. 1: Attachment.* London: Hogarth Press and the Institute of Psycho-analysis.

Bowlby, J. (1973). *Attachment and loss, Vol. 2: Separation: Anxiety and Anger.* London: Hogarth Press and the Institute of Psycho-analysis.

Briere, J. (2002). Treating adult survivors of severe childhood abuse and neglect: Further development of an integrative model. In J. E. B. Myers, L. Berliner, J. Briere, C. T. Hendrix, T. Reid, & C. Jenny (Eds.), *The APSAC handbook on child maltreatment* (2nd ed., pp. 175–203). Newbury Park, CA: Sage.

Briere, J., & Scott, C. (2015). *Principles of trauma therapy: A guide to symptoms, evaluation, and treatment, DSM-5 update* (2nd ed.). Thousand Oaks, CA: Sage.

Calhoun, L. G., & Tedeschi, R. G. (2006a). The foundations of posttraumatic growth: A expanded framework. In L. G. Calhoun & R. G. Tedeschi (Eds.), *Handbook of posttraumatic growth: Research and Practice* (pp. 3–23). New York: Lawrence Erlbaum Associates.

Calhoun, L. G., & Tedeschi, R. G. (Eds.). (2006b). *Handbook of posttraumatic growth: Research and practice*. New York: Lawrence Erlbaum Associates.

Courtois, C. A., & Ford, J. D. (Eds.). (2013). *Treating complex traumatic stress disorders: Scientific foundations and therapeutic models*. New York: The Guilford Press.

Davis, C. G., & Nolen-Hoeksema, S. (2001). Loss and meaning: How do people make sense of loss? *American Behavioral Scientist, 44*(5), 726–741.

Davis, C. G., Nolen-Hoeksema, S., & Larson, J. (1998). Making sense of loss and benefiting from the experience: Two construals of meaning. *Journal of Personality and Social Psychology, 75*(2), 561–574.

Davis, C. G., Wortman, C. B., Lehman, D. R., & Silver, R. C. (2000). Searching for meaning in loss: Are clinical assumptions correct? *Death Studies, 24*, 497–540.

Erikson, E. (1968). *Identity: Youth and crisis*. New York: Norton.

Ford, J. D., Grasso, D. J., Elhai, J. D., & Courtois, C. A. (2015). *Posttraumatic stress disorder: Scientific and professional dimensions* (2nd ed.). San Diego, CA: Elsevier Academic Press.

Frankl, V. E. (1946/1984). *Man's search for meaning*. New York: Washington Square Press.

Fullerton, C. (2004). Shared meaning following trauma: Bridging generations and cultures. *Psychiatry, 67*(1), 61–62.

Hecker, T., Hermenau, K., Crombach, A., & Elbert, T. (2015). Treating traumatized offenders and veterans by means of narrative exposure therapy. *Frontiers in Psychiatry, 6*.

Hunt, N., & McHale, S. (2008). Memory and meaning: Individual and social aspects of memory narratives. *Journal of Loss and Trauma, 13*(1), 42–58. https://doi.org/10.1080/15325020701296851

Hyden, L. C., & Brockmeier, J. (Eds.). (2008). *Health, illness and culture: Broken narratives*. New York: Routledge.

Janoff-Bulman, R. (1992). *Shattered assumptions: Towards a new psychology of trauma*. New York: The Free Press.

Janoff-Bulman, R. (2006). Schema-change perspectives on posttraumatic growth. In L. G. Calhoun & R. G. Tedeschi (Eds.), *Handbook of posttraumatic growth: Research and practice* (pp. 81–99). New York: Lawrence Erlbaum Associates.

Kitch, C. (2003). Mourning in America: Ritual, redemption, and recovery in new narrative after September 11. *Journalism Studies, 4*(2), 213–224.

Ladegaard, H. J. (2015). Coping with trauma in domestic migrant worker narratives: Linguistic, emotional and psychological perspectives. *Journal of SocioLinguistics, 19*(2), 189–221. https://doi.org/10.1111/josl.12117

MacManus, D., Rona, R., Dickson, H., Somaini, G., Fear, N., & Wessely, S. (2015). Aggressive and violent behavior among military personnel deployed to Iraq and Afghanistan: Prevalence and link with deployment and combat exposure. *Epidemiologic Reviews, 37*(1), 196–212. https://doi.org/10.1093/epirev/mxu006

McTighe, J. P., & Tosone, C. (2015). Narrative and meaning-making among Manhattan social workers in the wake of September 11, 2001. *Social Work in Mental Health, 13*(4), 299–317. https://doi.org/10.1080/15332985.2014.977420

Neimeyer, R. A. (2001a). The language of loss: Grief therapy as a process of meaning reconstruction. In R. A. Neimeyer (Ed.), *Meaning reconstruction and the experience of loss* (pp. 261–292). Washington, DC: American Psychological Association.

Neimeyer, R. A. (Ed.). (2001b). *Meaning reconstruction and the experience of loss*. Washington, DC: American Psychological Association.

Neimeyer, R. A. (2004). Fostering posttraumatic growth: A narrative contribution. *Psychological Inquiry, 15*(53–59).

References

Neimeyer, R. A. (2005). Tragedy and transformation: Meaning reconstruction in the wake of traumatic loss. In S. Heilman (Ed.), *Death, bereavement, and mourning*. New Brunswick: Transaction Publishers.

Neimeyer, R. A. (2006). Re-storying loss: Fostering growth in the posttraumatic narrative. In L. G. Calhoun & R. G. Tedeschi (Eds.), *Handbook of posttraumatic growth: Research and practice* (pp. 68–80). New York: Lawrence Erlbaum Associates.

Newman, E., Briere, J., & Kirlic, N. (2012). Clinical assessment as a form of listening and intervention. In R. A. McMackin, E. Newman, J. M. Fogler, & T. M. Keane (Eds.), *Trauma therapy in context: The science and craft of evidence-based practice* (pp. 51–71). Washington, DC: American Psychological Association.

Park, C. L., & Folkman, S. (1997). Meaning in the context of stress and coping. *Review of General Psychology, 1*(2), 115–144.

Ramchand, R., Rudavsky, R., Grant, S., Tanielian, T., & Joycox, L. (2015). Prevalence of, risk factors for, and consequences of posttraumatic stress disorder and other mental health problems in military populations deployed to Iraq and Afghanistan. *Current PsySchiatric Reports, 17*(5), 1–11. https://doi.org/10.1007/s11920-015-0575-z

Rennicke, C. (2007). *Searching for meaning of the September 11, 2001 World Trade Center Attack and its impact on mental health outcomes among high exposure survivors in New York City*. (Dissertation), Columbia University.

Riessman, C. K. (2008). *Narrative methods for the human sciences*. Thousand Oaks, CA: Sage.

Shane, L., & Kime, P. (2016, July 7). New VA study finds 20 veterans commit suicide each day. *Military Times*. Retrieved from https://www.militarytimes.com/veterans/2016/07/07/new-va-study-finds-20-veterans-commit-suicide-each-day/.

Shohet, M. (2007). Narrating anorexia: "Full" and "struggling" genres of recovery. *Ethos, 35*, 344–382.

Stern, D. N. (1985). *The interpersonal world of the human infant: A view from psychoanalysis and developmental psychology*. New York: Basic Books.

Tedeschi, R. G., & Calhoun, L. G. (1995). *Trauma & transformation: Growing in the aftermath of suffering*. Thousand Oaks, CA: Sage.

Tedeschi, R. G., & Calhoun, L. G. (2004). Posttraumatic growth: Conceptual foundations and empirical evidence. *Psychological Inquiry, 15*, 1–18.

van der Kolk, B. A. (2014). *The body keeps the score: Brain, mind, and body in the healing of trauma*. New York: Viking.

Winnicott, D. W. (1965). *The maturational process and the facilitating environment*. New York: International Universities Press.

Yehuda, R., Daskalakis, N. P., Bierer, L. M., Bader, H. N., Klengel, T., Holsboer, F., & Binder, E. B. (2016). Holocaust exposure induced intergenerational effects on FKBP5 methylation. *Biological Psychiatry, 80*(5), 372–380. https://doi.org/10.1016/j.biopsych.2015.08.005

Chapter 4
Spiritual Stories: Exploring Ultimate Meaning in Social Work Practice

Guiding Questions

What do we mean by the term spirituality? How is this similar to and different from religion and religious beliefs?

What do we mean by spiritual narrative? How do narrative theory and practice help us engage clients' spiritual stories (and our own)?

What role does spiritual narrative have to play in clinical practice? Why is it important to attend to this in our work?

How is spirituality understood from the perspective of meaning making? What is the impact of this on our clients?

What is the relationship between the spiritual narratives of the client and the social worker? Why is it important for the social worker to understand their own spiritual narrative as they work with clients?

When you hear the word *spirituality* what feelings and images does it evoke in you? What about the word *religion*? Are they the same for you? Different? If so, how? Perhaps you associate one or the other of these words (or maybe both) with solace, connection, and a higher purpose in life. On the other hand, perhaps they suggest thoughts and feelings that are more negative? Spiritualty and religious experience are among the most intimate and personal aspects of life. They have the power to stir passionate reactions within us—both positive and negative. For many they are a source of great ambivalence. At the same time, research consistently finds that spirituality and religion—the beliefs and practices related to the experience of faith—are among the most robust and effective coping mechanisms that people who value them have for coping with adversity (Pargament, 2007; Pargament, Magyar-Russell, & Murray-Swank, 2005).

Spiritual narrative is the story that we tell of ultimate meaning, the meaning of our life and existence, indeed the meaning of life itself (Altmaier, 2013; Gockel, 2013; Pargament et al., 2005; Tuval-Mashiach & Dekel, 2014). For many, it is a story of relationship to a Higher Being, named in a variety of ways according to the traditions and beliefs in which we have been formed, who is the source and goal of our life. For others, the story takes on a variety of different forms. In this chapter we will consider the nature of spiritual narrative—the story of ultimate meaning that we tell in the most personal way as well as in social and communal ways. We will consider the nature of spirituality and religion—what they have in common and how they may be different. This will lead to an exploration of the role of spirituality and spiritual narrative in the treatment we offer and in the relationship we seek to develop with our clients. In keeping with this, we will cultivate an understanding of both the spirituality of the clients with whom we work and our own spirituality, since both of these impact the developing therapeutic relationship. Finally, we will examine some of the ways that we can effectively attend to spiritual narrative in the clinical situation.

So what do we mean by spirituality? How is it similar to or different from religion? If you examine the extensive literature in this area, you will come quickly to the conclusion that there are, indeed, numerous definitions of each of these terms. Fortunately, perhaps, there is a great deal of overlap in the way they are conceptualized. What is also somewhat helpful is that there seems to be near-universal agreement that it is important to understand the commonalities and differences between these two concepts (Canda & Furman, 2009; Cunningham, 2011; Pargament, 2007; Senreich, 2013).

For our purposes, we will operate from the perspective that spirituality is any attitude, practice, ritual, or belief system that orients me and my life to what is beyond me—what is, as I suggested above, *ultimate*. Spirituality is focused on connection. For its part, religion may be seen as a communal expression of belief in the Divine organized around a set of doctrines and practices that inform the living out of that belief system both in the community and in the world. Religion is focused on belonging.

It is important to notice the areas of overlap and distinction in these definitions. Can spirituality and religion fit together like hand and glove? They do in the lives of many. Is it possible, however, for the two to be more or less distinct? Yes. There is an increasing portion of the population that identifies as "spiritual but not religious" (Pew Research Center, 2014). This is an important dimension of experience and one that we will discuss at some length in this chapter.

Zinnbauer et al. (1997) examined what are now more commonly used distinctions by having study participants categorize themselves as religious and spiritual, religious but not spiritual, spiritual but not religious, or neither spiritual nor religious. For example, there are people who identify with a religious tradition, and who attend a house of worship affiliated with that tradition, but who do not *feel* a significant connection to God in their lives. Indeed some long for this kind of connection, while others will note that they attend for a sense of belonging to a community (which some would in fact think of as spiritual), for the moral guidance they receive, and even for the value of passing their religion on to their children.

It is also important to be aware that for many people who identify as "spiritual but not religious" the appeal of being part of a community is very real. To this end, we witness the increase in popularity of yoga studios (which for some is a form of exercise and for others is an exercise of spirualty) as well as meditation groups, centers, and classes. While not seeking to belong to a traditional religion, these individuals do value the sense of being on a journey together.

Even as we acknowledged the increasing commonality of identifying as "spiritual but not religious," Wong and Vinsky (2009) offer an important critique that is valuable for us as social workers to keep in mind. These authors suggest that the current "spiritual but not religious" distinction is the product of a Western, Eurocentric perspective and that individuals of many diverse backgrounds will not resonate with that division of spirituality and religiosity. They go on to caution that the "spiritual but not religious" point of view can inadvertently repeat and even further the marginalization and colonization of minority cultures. From this point of view, other cultures that identify more explicitly with religion may be subtly viewed as inferior, backwards, unenlightened, or naïve in their traditional beliefs. In keeping with this, social workers need to be attentive to the possibility of viewing clients of any background who hold more traditional religious beliefs, whether these are familiar to the social worker or not, as curious, quaint, or somehow uncritical in their thinking and approach to life.

As you read this, you may get the sense that there could be nearly endless permutations to the relationship between spirituality and religion. I would suggest that is quite accurate. So how do we get our minds around this? Do we need to? Pargament (2007) suggests that what ties it all together is the search for *the sacred*. Though there are both commonalities and differences in what we mean by the sacred, for most people it involves attention to what I have referred to as *the ultimate*—the infinite horizon that frames the experience of being human and has us continually reaching beyond ourselves for a deeper and deeper sense of meaning. That kind of meaning may be truly ineffable to us on some level. But when we seek to engage each other in that journey, when we seek to talk with each other about our experience of that journey, we do so again and again in story.

For us as clinicians, this kind of understanding is essential if we are to attend to and be part of the crafting of the client's spiritual narrative. As we will see, addressing the spiritual narrative in treatment is not about placing ourselves in the position of pastor, rabbi, imam, guru, or any other spiritual leader (Canda & Furman, 2009). It is not about our comprehensive knowledge of all things spiritual and religious (though a developing base of general knowledge can be somewhat helpful). It is about our ability to sit with, be open to, and wonder about to a key area of the diversity of our clients—one that, for many, has enormous meaning (Oxhandler & Pargament, 2014; Oxhandler, Parrish, Torres, & Achenbaum, 2015). It is our willingness to ask the question about the role of spirituality in their life, to listen to their spiritual narrative, and to be open to what we hear. That may seem like a tall order, and in fact it may be. So let's see how we can get there.

First of all, we might begin with an understanding of why this matters. Even in what many consider to be an increasingly secularized society, 80% of US adults continue to view religion as "somewhat important" and 58% view it as "very important." This is true even among those whose religion or spirituality takes a more individualized and less traditional form (Pew Forum on Religion and Public Life, 2012, October 9). Furthermore, data consistently show that integration of religious and spiritual experience and perspectives into psychotherapy has positive effects on outcomes (Oxhandler & Pargament, 2014; Pargament, 1997). Clients even report that they would like their spirituality and religion to be incorporated into the work they do with their therapist, though findings suggest that they are very commonly not even asked about it (Oxhandler & Pargament, 2014).

When I teach about this in class, I notice that there is often still a reticence on the part of many students to talk about spirituality (Northcut, 2004; Oxhandler et al., 2015). My challenge to them is to ask themselves if there is any other aspect of their clients' experience that was meaningful to them that they would not want to know about. The answer is consistently *no*. Of course we want to know the story of our clients' experience of race and ethnicity. Of course we want to know about the story of their sexuality or any traumas they have experienced in life. Why then, I ask, would the story of their spirituality or religious faith be different? This is particularly true, I suggest, when we note that research consistently finds that spirituality is among the most effective coping mechanisms that our clients have for coping with adversity, and a means of re-appraising and reframing their experience in a greater context (Pargament, 2007). That ability commonly provides a sense of mastery and control in the face of difficult circumstances (Hodge, 2015).

The spiritual narrative has everything to do with how our clients make meaning of the world and of their existence, and therein lies its importance. Attention to this part of their narrative signals an awareness and a readiness on our part to take seriously the whole of their personhood and what is meaningful to them. In this sense, one might note how the very act of inquiring about spirituality and what it means to our client may be viewed as an intervention (Hodge, 2015). Some will say that they do not experience spirituality or religion as salient in their life, and that is of course fine. However, inasmuch as that relationship to the sacred or the ultimate is important to them, the integration of clients' spiritual narrative can have a powerful impact on the therapeutic space that we create together.

Like many aspects of our client's story, their spiritual narrative may well not resemble ours, something we will explore in greater depth later in this chapter. Nor does it need to. We know that, in order for us to work effectively with clients, it is not important that we be "like" them. What is important is not commonality, but understanding, and a respect for the value of their story.

I once had the opportunity to do some work in a large children's hospital. Specifically, I worked on the neurosurgery and orthopedics unit. The children, from preschool age through adolescence, were commonly hospitalized because of brain tumors and other conditions like Spina Bifida. One day, as I was making rounds on the unit, I knocked gently on a partially closed door. The lights had been dimmed in the room. A woman's voice invited me in. I met a mother whose name I no longer remember. But I do remember our time together. I introduced myself and tried to see if I could be helpful to her in some way. She and her husband had immigrated to the United States from India some years earlier. She brought me to the bedside of her son who was napping. He was 6 years old and was scheduled to have a brain tumor removed the following morning. She told me how terrified she was and how she was clinging to her faith, praying that he would be well. I asked what her faith was and she told me she was Baha'i. I had heard of Baha'i, but to be truthful I did not know much of anything about it. So I asked her if there was anything in particular that her faith said about how to cope with fear and suffering, any prayers or rituals? She said that yes, there was a common prayer, a song in fact, that one could sing in times of doubt and fear. It spoke of God's goodness and the way God takes care of us all. She had been praying it throughout the day as she kept watch over her son. I asked if I could hear it. She smiled and took my hand. She closed her eyes and began to sing in a language, the name of which I did not even know, words I could not understand. But it didn't matter. All that mattered was presence—holding her hand, standing by the bedside of her son while she managed her fear and vulnerability in the best, most powerful way she knew how. It was a beautiful song, and the peace that it brought her was apparent. When she finished the prayer she hugged me and thanked me for praying with her. Spiritual narrative invites us to enter into the way our clients make meaning of some of their greatest, most ultimate concerns.

The Formation of Spiritual Narratives: Individual, Communal, and Social

In Chap. 1 we considered the fact that our narratives and the narrative structure of our living are not solely the products of our own internal life. Rather, we noted, we are shaped by the communal and social contexts in which we live and grow. The storytelling of the world around us comes to shape the way we see the world and the range of understandings or interpretations we make of it (Bruner, 1990, 1991). The more life experience we get, the more diversity we are exposed to, the more nuanced will be the palette of interpretive possibilities at our disposal in the formation of our narratives. The same is true with respect to spiritual narrative.

Let us consider for example the notion of the image of God. How do we arrive at an image of God? This is particularly important to consider for those who endorse a theistic faith—one founded on the belief in the existence of God. I would suggest, however, that if the very word *God* has any meaning to you at all—even just semantically, then the "image of God" construct has meaning for you as well. Even a professed atheist, for example, can have an image of the God in whom he or she does not believe.

So where does that image come from? The mind readily and correctly turns to answers such as culture, society, tradition, and the religious faith one was exposed to as a child. We might consider, however, that there is more to it than that. On the deepest, most internalized level, the image of God is rooted in our earliest life experience and the formative relationship we have to the most significant people in our life (Rizzuto, 1974, 1979). For most of us this is likely mother and father. For others it may be a different caretaker who stands as that earliest and most important attachment figure. These most significant experiences result in what Hall (2004) refers to as implicit relational representations—deep learnings about others and the world that may not emerge as clearly formulated thoughts, but nonetheless shape our sense of self, others, and relationships in the world.

When we are eventually introduced to the idea of God and the possibility of a relationship to God, these first formative figures and our implicit relational representations serve as the experiential template for the propositions we learn about God's nature, identity, and view of the world and us (Rizzuto, 1974, 1979). By extension, this also impacts our subsequent experience of self and relationships in the world (Carlson & Erickson, 2000). For example, consider a child learning that God loves and cares for her—like a mother or father loves their daughter—but even more so. What has been that child's experience of love from mother and father (or mother/father figure)? Has the child had an experience, albeit imperfect, of being loved, seen, understood, valued, forgiven when necessary, held, cherished, seen as a source of delight …? Or has that child been told verbally or nonverbally that she is unworthy, unwanted, cast aside, in the way …? The child who goes on to learn about a God who is the ultimate parent, the supreme caretaker, the one whose loving gaze never wanders and whose hand never fails to support and sustain, may find in this a felt extension of the love they have already experienced, or a metaphor that is exceedingly hard to grasp in the absence of any real-world experience with which to compare it.

A young woman I once worked with came to see me initially reporting that she thought she might have bipolar disorder. Her father was diagnosed with the mood disorder when he was in his early 20s and she felt there was reason to suspect she suffered from the condition as well. This intrigued me since there was no objective evidence for that conclusion. In fact, she did not endorse any of the defining symptoms of bipolar disorder. Yet she clearly wanted to be in treatment. So we began. We met every week for 2 years before she was finally able to disclose to me, gradually and with enormous pain, the reason she had begun treatment with me in the first place. The week prior to her first call to me to begin therapy, she was sitting in Church and had begun having flashbacks: scenes and images from her adolescence, things so awful they shook her to her core. As if a floodgate had opened, and for reasons she did not understand, she began to remember the experience of being sexually abused by her father.

Her mother worked long hours at a high-level corporate job while her father, due to his unstable mental health, had not held a steady job for years. This left her home alone with him typically every day after school and often long into the evening. This was when the abuse took place. She did not remember exactly when it began although she had vivid recall of what she thought was the first episode of the abuse itself. Though she was convinced that it continued for at least a couple of years, she could not recall exactly how or why it stopped.

I tell this story in the context of this chapter because of an experience she had that neither of us expected. You will recall that she had her first flashback while she was in Church. Though she was raised as nominally religious in a Protestant family, they did not attend Church. In her young adulthood, she became interested in matters of faith and felt herself drawn to Church. She found a group for Christian Young Adults and began to attend weekly. Eventually, this led her to find a Church of her own. After some time, she made the decision to become Catholic. Though she maintained distance from her parents with whom she had an ambivalent relationship, her mother attended her Confirmation and this was very meaningful to her. All in all, her experience of faith had been deeply life giving. She found a great sense of meaning in her belief and in the warmth of a community of faith.

She and I continued to work together for a few more years on her experience of trauma and its consequences, as well as helping her negotiate a number of other hurdles appropriate to her stage of life. The end of our work drew near when she decided to relocate to another state for a job opportunity. We spent some time reflecting on the journey she had taken in treatment and what it meant to her. After working together for so long, I knew that we had a deep therapeutic alliance and that she felt close to me. We had talked often of her growing spirituality and experience of faith. But I was nonetheless surprised by what she shared with me. She said that as much as faith and her relationship to God meant to her, the one thing she had never been able to connect with emotionally, even prior to regaining an awareness of the abuse of her childhood, was the experience of God as a father. She grasped the idea intellectually, she said. But it never spoke to her or meant anything to her personally—until she met me. Her relationship with me, she said, helped her to understand what it was like to be safe and protected, seen and cared for by a man. I was that father figure for her. It was a powerful moment for us both, a moment that reminded me of the sacredness of the relationship we develop with our clients and of the awesome ways it can shape our narratives and us, even beyond our own expectations.

It is also true to say that for some individuals, the experience of faith in a loving God may serve as a counterpoint to a disappointing reality of relationships in the world. With our sometimes stunning ability to overcome adversity, our futures are not once and for all determined by the shortcomings of our earliest caregivers. Though we bear within us the scars that result from our pain, and though we as social workers do not have the power to give someone a different past, many people exhibit an almost heroic capacity to overcome and to experience love.

A number of scholars have explored the implications of narrative for an understanding of the role of spirituality and a relationship to God in the development of one's sense of self. Carlson and Erikson (2000), for example, have noted that for many people, God is the most significant person in their religious and spiritual life, making the quality of this relationship highly salient. Taking an approach drawn from the work of White (2007; White & Epston, 1990), they encourage exploring the client's perception of how God thinks of and sees them as a person. This is meant to reveal not only something of the person's sense of self in the eyes of God, but also their view of the state of that relationship. Those clients for whom that relationship and image are strong and affirming have touched upon a resource that may be of great benefit in their therapeutic work.

For others, however, this may not be the case. When the exploration of this story reveals a relationship that is limiting or disempowering, the authors suggest White's narrative approach to re-author that story using the techniques of deconstruction questions, externalizing language, and searching for exceptions. By examining, for example, the impact that depression has had on the client's image of God (e.g., externalizing and deconstructing the belief that I am unlovable and God doesn't care about me), they suggest that the God image and the client's relationship to God may be reconstructed. This is aided by the exploration of exceptions to this rule (e.g., "Was there ever a time that you felt loved or blessed by God? Tell me about that time? What made it different?"). Carlson and Erikson suggest that this is one way of liberating the relationship to God from a disempowering narrative that may negatively impact the client's sense of self.

In a similar vein, Olson et al. (2016) have examined the use of God Image Narrative Therapy for fostering increased coherence in both God and life narratives of clients. Drawing on the work of Rizzuto (1979), they note the distinction between *God concept* (beliefs and conceptual propositions about God) and *God image* (shaped by an affective experience of God and informed by the implicit relational representations discussed earlier). Based on the belief that a healthy spirituality is marked by a high degree of integration between God concept and God image, when the relational experiences that inform the God image result in a lack of congruence with one's God concept, internal conflict will result. The authors suggest that narrative interventions such as journal writing hold promise for increasing that level of coherence and fostering an improved relationship to God.

In addition to our earliest significant relationships, it is also important to acknowledge that our spiritual narrative is shaped by the social and historical context in which we live. Some of us have grown up in communities and social worlds where we rarely encountered anyone different from ourselves. Others encountered a great deal of diversity. This is as true of spirituality as it is of politics, race, sexuality, or any other dimension of life. I recall as a boy growing up in Brooklyn, sitting by the open window of our apartment on a hot summer night, straining to catch a breeze while listening to the cadence of the Latino Pentecostal preacher praying loudly into his microphone in a language I didn't understand from the storefront church on my corner. I remember walking a few blocks on a Sunday afternoon with my parents to go shopping on 13th avenue, a largely Hasidic Jewish neighborhood where I passed booths constructed on balconies for Succoth, saw boys my own age dressed so differently from me, groups of men and women speaking yet another language I didn't understand, and feeling like the outsider in a cultural and spiritual world so different from my own.

Meaning making through spiritual narrative, then, does not just happen on individual levels, but on communal levels as well. In this sense, the narrative of the individual is embedded in the narrative of the community in which it finds a sense of identity (MacIntyre, 1985). Not surprisingly, this is particularly true in contexts that tend to more collectivistic than individualistic (e.g., Asian, Middle Eastern, and African cultures). Among these groups, when religion is highly salient to the life of the community, it is more frequently and consistently turned to as a means of coping (Pargament, 1997; Tuval-Mashiach & Dekel, 2014).

Our spiritual identity takes on social and political overtones as well. It is almost a cliché at this point to comment that many of the bloodiest wars in history have been fought in the name of God, and in the perceived defense of a set of beliefs. In ways that reach back as far as the Biblical scapegoat itself (Lev.16: 20–22), we project onto the other all badness so as to imagine ourselves innocent and justified (Volkan, 1988). In our day, we see this unfold around the world. We have debates over whether or not the United States is a Christian nation. Our fear of the other manifests in forms both old and new, as with Islamophobia when we confuse the tenets of a peaceful religion for the terror perpetrated by a few under the supposed guise of faith. We fight generation after generation over which religious group has the most legitimate claim to land considered sacred by them all.

Among major religious groups (e.g., Judaism, Islam, Christianity) there has always been ongoing debate as to what it means to live faith and spirituality authentically. Some of this, no doubt, is the product of genuine inquiry and the desire to live faith wholeheartedly. It emerges from our search for the communal narrative that speaks to us as an expression of faith and a path toward the spiritual life we seek. However, this instinct has also at times been born from the wish to cling to righteousness while repudiating the other. In those moments, it has served less the spiritual interests of human beings and more their self-interest.

When considering the role of spiritual narrative, it is also important to address the negative role that religion and faith have played in the lives of many people. As social workers, when we inquire about our clients' sense of spirituality, we must acknowledge that many feel no attraction to religious and spiritual groups because of these very issues. Additionally, we will often enough encounter those who have felt harshly judged by the religious communities to which they belong (even nominally) or that they would never be considered worthy of belonging because of some aspect of their life. When these issues are significant to our clients, it can be important to understand something of the actual teachings of their faith tradition, since even members of a faith community often have less than a full understanding of the doctrines of the group. At other times, of course, there is an actual disconnect between the beliefs of the individual and those of a religious organization that results in a poor fit. At still other, increasingly common times, the relationship between the individual and the community is marked by ambivalence. In these instances, people may remain affiliated with their religious community, but find their own comfortable balance between distance and closeness in which they hold on to what is most meaningful while often rejecting the rest.

I once worked with a young woman in her late teens who had come to see me to talk about some issues that were concerning her in her relationships. While these issues caused her some distress, she was otherwise high functioning, well adjusted, and apparently happy. She had mentioned during assessment that she was very religious and had for a number of years participated regularly in the youth group at her Catholic Church. I was rather startled then, when several months into our work together, she commented in the midst of a broader discussion about an unrelated topic, "Well, I guess it doesn't matter since I'm going to hell anyway." When I asked her what she meant, she grew quiet and tearful. She shared with me that she had had an abortion when she was in high school. She felt deeply conflicted and guilty about it still and, while superficially content with her life, carried with her a sense that no matter what she did in life, she would be punished for that choice.

Shortly after the abortion, she went to confession and sincerely sought forgiveness as her tradition had taught her to do. But in her mind, that didn't matter. Even though she had received absolution, it was not enough to alter her fate. For all the time we had spent working on the relationship issues so typical of her stage of development, there we sat with the greatest heaviness of her heart laid bare. Sensing that this was a time when the input of a member of the clergy might be useful, I asked her if she had ever talked about this with her pastor to whom she was close. She had not, but readily accepted my suggestion that she do so.

When I saw her the following week, she told me about what a powerful experience that had been. Not only had the pastor been deeply kind and compassionate, she said. He also assured her that it was not at all part of her faith tradition that she was doomed to be separated from God forever. His words were of enormous comfort to her and changed not only her view of her place in her religious community, but also her sense of self. This was an instance where the ability to refer to a trusted member of the clergy was of great importance in that her pastor was invested with the moral and personal authority to provide her a kind of reassurance that would not come readily from anywhere else (Pargament, 2007).

I realize, of course, that this story of success could be countered by others that did not go as well. I have heard of many interactions with religious figures who were harsh and condemning, whether this represented the authentic teachings of their faith or not. Additionally, we should also note that when our clients' struggles evoke guilt or some other form of inner conflict, the care of even the most trusted and compassionate member of the clergy may not be enough to assuage the turmoil they feel (Albertsen, O'Connor, & Berry, 2006; McCullough, Pargament, & Thoresen, 2000). These narratives can be so complex and so deeply embedded that they may only yield, or even become more pliable, after much repeated but gentle work with a skilled and empathic clinician.

When we are working with narratives that are so woven into the fabric of our sense of self, change will often only happen gradually over time. It seems to me that it is instinctual for us to want to deal with a problem "once and for all" and then "move on." I have sat with many clients who have found themselves discouraged by the fact that they are returning to issues they thought they had "dealt with" years before. They believed this or that part of their story was behind them and would resurface no more. This itself is a narrative.

There are two images that I have found helpful in these moments. One is that people tend to think of their experience in linear fashion. I have made progress from here to there, and so if I find myself dealing with an issue from the so-called past, it means that I have moved backwards or lost ground; I have failed somehow. My sense of it, however, is that our life course is more like a spiral. Picture it. We can indeed move along and yet in some respect we may find ourselves returning again and again to the same places, even if not in the same way.

The second image is of geological fault lines. Recall learning in science class that where the earth's tectonic plates come together the planet is vulnerable to earthquakes. Things may remain quiet and stable for long periods of time, even by geological standards. But if there is going to be some unrest, it will most assuredly occur along that fault line. Our lives are much the same way. We rightly invest time and energy tending to the wounds that life has inflicted upon us in one way or another. We pursue the healing that we know we need. But it is also true that these are our tender and vulnerable places, the areas that are most likely to be triggered when life is hard and the road we walk seems most difficult. However, this is not a reason to despair. Instead, I believe it is a call to know and understand our story even more deeply, to embrace it and extend to ourselves the kind of compassion we need but may never have gotten, at least in sufficient measure. And that can be a mighty challenge.

For some individuals, it is also true that a negative experience of spirituality comes not from a particular issue around which they experience conflict, but from a more fundamental sense of the worthiness of their own existence. Note that some have had an experience of religion that they felt simply told them they were bad. For others, their sense of badness finds a lightening rod of confirmation in religion. It is important to understand the extent to which the client has bought into that message about badness and perhaps the factors that might have facilitated that. As we discussed earlier, the image of God is born, at least in part, from the nature of the significant early relationships in our lives. When these have been toxic or in some way damaging to a healthy sense of self, then seeing my badness reflected cosmically in the face of God is much more likely (Gurney & Rogers, 2007; Hall, 2007; Rizzuto, 1974). In my experience, this results in a deeply held narrative that takes a good deal of time and patience to work with.

How then might we assess the quality of a person's spiritual narrative? I suggest that as we listen deeply and begin to hear and understand their story, we tune in to whether that narrative is supportive or conflictual. Does it enhance or detract from their functioning? This requires listening not on a surface level, but to the deeper meaning that their spirituality has for them and the way they view themselves.

The Spirituality and Spiritual Narrative of the Social Worker and Its Role in Treatment

It is also essential that we consider the spirituality and spiritual narrative of the social worker and the role this may play in treatment. Historically, we know, there has been reluctance on the part of many social workers to "go there" when it comes to issues of spirituality and religion. For some, this aversion to the topic of spirituality no doubt continues, though there is evidence that this is changing (Oxhandler et al., 2015). Even when we know that clients overwhelmingly affirm that they would like their spirituality to be incorporated into their treatment, many social workers still hold back (Hodge & Horvath, 2011; Lietz & Hodge, 2013; Northcut, 2000; Oxhandler & Pargament, 2014; Oxhandler et al., 2015; Stanley et al., 2011). I have heard social workers say things like "Well, that doesn't apply to my work. That has nothing to do with my role." My strong sense has been that this is related less to a philosophical position on the scope of the social worker's role and more to hesitation to venture into territory that seems foreign. Even social workers who report a good deal of self-efficacy when it comes to addressing spirituality report that they do not necessarily do so consistently (Oxhandler et al., 2015). As I suggested above, it is certainly wise and appropriate to refer a client to a member of the clergy or some other representative of a religious faith when spiritual questions are primary. But as we've seen, the deep sense of meaning that we connect with religion and spirituality makes it important to the clinical work we do with clients.

This history of antipathy between the mental health professions and religion or spirituality certainly dates back to the life and work of Freud and his social and intellectual milieu, as well as the relationship he had to the religion of his own upbringing (Bingaman, 2003; Gay, 2006; Northcut, 2004). In the world of psychoanalysis, the legacy of rejection of all things religious and the insistence that faith is a neurosis to be worked through has certainly evolved in the century since Freud was developing his ideas. The same is true in the field of social work and the other mental health disciplines. Not only has there been an increasing volume of research that looks at religion and spirituality as key variables, but the standards governing social work education and the code of ethics by which we practice reflect this change as well. The 2015 Educational Policy and Accreditation Standards of the Council on Social Work Education (Council on Social Work Education, 2015), for example, address religion and spirituality as a dimension of diversity both in Competency 2 and Educational Policy 3.0. Similarly, the Code of Ethics of the National Association of Social Workers (2008) mandates that social workers take into consideration the impact of clients' religious beliefs and practices as well as their own when making ethical decisions, and avoid conflicts of interest in this regard.

So when we think about attending to the spiritual narratives of our clients, how do we begin? As I have suggested, perhaps the best starting place is an attention to spirituality and religion as an element of diversity just like any other. Social workers do an outstanding job of maintaining a respectful awareness of the importance and value of diversity of all its forms. Built into our curriculum and professional orientation is an attunement not only to the diversity of the client but our own as well. And when you and the client come together, something even greater can emerge.

In order for this to happen, however, we need to be self-aware (Northcut, 2000, 2004). This entails cultivating a sense of the role of religion and spirituality in our own lives. As much as we talk about attending to the role of spiritual stories in the lives of our clients we need to attend to our own as well—whatever they may be. And just as spiritual stories are often a source of coping and meaning making for clients, so too they may be for us. Social workers are continually exposed to the struggles of others in a way that can challenge our own meaning making. We are increasingly well trained in the risks of secondary trauma, vicarious traumatization, and shared trauma (Figley, 1995; McCann & Pearlman, 1990; Naturale, 2007; Pearlman & Saakvitne, 1995; Tosone, McTighe, & Bauwens, 2015; Tosone, McTighe, Bauwens, & Naturale, 2011). For those of us who are engaged in the care of others, our own spiritual resources can serve as an important means of self-care in the face of these personal and professional stressors (Martis & Westhues, 2015).

Additionally, we need to know our own narrative so that we can use it mindfully and purposefully for the benefit of the client. We need to know not only who we are and how we got here, but also what we know and what we don't know. We can ask ourselves, "Was I raised in a spiritual framework that informed my sense of identity, life, and the world? What has been that spiritual narrative for me and how has it evolved? Does it feel positive, neutral, negative? Have I experienced my spiritual narrative as life giving, alienating, ambivalent? In what ways? Can I contain my story and the experiences that inform it in order to allow the client's narrative to be her own?" This reflective self-awareness can then allow us to listen to our clients and their spiritual story and ask ourselves key questions like "How does this story contribute to my client's sense of self and the meaning of life and the world? How important is this story to his or her meaning making? Is their spiritual story a helpful resource in their coping? Is it a stumbling block or obstacle? Is it both?"

In the end, if we wish to take seriously the spiritual and religious narratives of our clients and to integrate those as potentially powerful resources in their work of healing and growth, I suggest that there are a few things to which we might attend. First, we will benefit from knowing ourselves and our own spiritual story in all of its complexity. This will help us be more available to our clients. Next, we can do our best to expand our grasp of the meaning and functions of the spiritual story—our own and others'. This work can be undertaken in the social work classroom for sure (Barker & Floersch, 2010; Northcut, 2004; Senreich, 2013), but like other areas of professional development, it needs to be nurtured and sustained over the course of our professional life. Finally, we can ask our clients. We can listen for fragmented or subjugated narratives, explore a new tradition, consider someone else's point of view, notice and suspend the judgment that comes from conflicting narratives, and contain them. Taking a religious and spiritual history validates it as something important and signals to the client our own openness to hearing and incorporating this part of their story (Canda & Furman, 2009; Hodge, 2015; Northcut, 2000; Pargament, 2007). The challenge is then, of course, to actually *be* open. Remember that you can always refer to an "expert" such as a member of the clergy if necessary, and supervision or other professional consultation is a potential source of support. But don't lose sight of the fact that in the end, you are listening to the way your client makes meaning—ultimate meaning—of their life and experience. I suggest that nothing could be more pertinent to the work we do.

Case Example

Colleen was a woman in her late 30s who came to see me for help managing the great deal of stress she experienced in her daily life. She was married and, though she loved her husband, there was a fair degree of arguing and tension in the house, mostly resulting from what seemed like the never-ending flow of chores, errands, and responsibilities they shared. In some senses, they lived a very traditional life. He worked hard at a blue-collar job with long hours. She was a part-time graduate student and part-time worker. She shouldered the lion's share of the responsibility for managing the day-to-day needs of their home and their three school-aged children, including cooking, cleaning, and playing chauffeur to school, games, and other activities. They didn't have a lot of money but they were managing to get by. Colleen and her husband didn't get to spend much time alone together, but they tried here and there, knowing that it was important, and they enjoyed each other's company. They even managed to sustain a mostly satisfying, if somewhat rushed sex life.

In therapy, Colleen was able to voice a genuine appreciation for what they had in life and she saw goodness in it. But she also felt deeply stressed, and with that stress came a weariness that was unsettling, not just because of the emotion itself, but because she didn't want to feel that way about her life. This led us in session to explore two particular themes in her narrative: the ways she coped with stress and the meaning she made of her life and circumstances. Colleen struggled with these. The main coping skill she was able to identify was simply holding on and not giving up. "You just get through it," she would say. She talked about possibly going to the gym or trying to get together with her friends more often, but these felt like more reflexive responses, the kind of thing you're supposed to say. Isn't that what people do to cope? Where would she even get time for that? It felt like just one more thing to do. As for meaning, she felt at a loss. What *did* it all mean really?

> We sat with these questions for some time in session. Eventually, I asked Colleen, "Do you consider yourself to be a spiritual or religious person?" Her face revealed a mixture of surprise and curiosity.
> "Definitely! I am a very religious person. Why?"
> "Tell me about your faith? What does it mean to you?"
> "Well, it means everything. I've always been a religious person. I was raised Methodist, but we've been going to the same Church together every week for the past 12 years. It's sort of non-denominational Christian, but I've never had such an experience of loving Church before, of feeling like I belong."
> "What is it about your Church that makes that so?"
> "Well… I guess it's the community. There's a lot of support there. We have really good friends who go there too. There's the preaching, the music, the teaching… I guess there's a whole lot. But when I think about it, I think what is most important is that I learned to pray there. It's where I developed a real relationship to God. I feel like I got to know more about who God is there. I feel loved there."
> "That's very powerful, "I said. "What is it like for you to be talking about this with me?"
> Colleen chuckled and again looked puzzled. "You know what's funny? I didn't think I was allowed to talk about that here."
> "Really? Where do you think that feeling comes from? Does it feel like something I conveyed to you?"
> "No. Not really. I guess it's just that, I've been in therapy before and no one has ever asked about it. Plus, I don't know, you sort of get this impression that faith is faith, and therapy is therapy. I guess I don't know where that comes from."
> "Well it seems to me that your faith, your spirituality is deeply important to you. It's a really important part of the story of your life, of who you are. And knowing that there is so much about life that is also really stressful, maybe we should pay attention to your spirituality, listen to it. What do you think?"
> "I think that would be great."

Colleen went on to talk more about her spirituality and to make more explicit connections between her faith and the way she handled life's stress. She talked about her prayer life and her desire to be part of the prayer group at her Church, something that she thought she really could fit into her schedule since it took place while her children were in Sunday school. She identified that prayer was perhaps her most important coping mechanism, and that her faith not only gave her guidance about how she should live her life and the choices she should make, but also provided her with an understanding of what she was doing it all for. We continued to work in therapy on communication with her husband, handling the concerns she had for her kids, developing other stress management strategies, and so on. But the acknowledgement and inclusion of her faith and spirituality became a current that ran through the whole of our work. Now that it was on the table and something she knew she could talk about, Colleen came back again and again to her spirituality and how she was using it to manage stress and make sense of her life.

From a distinctly narrative perspective, Colleen and I were working on two levels. First, we were exploring the narrative of her spirituality and its significance for the way she managed stress and the challenges of life. Colleen articulated a narrative of belonging, of feeling loved by God, family, and community, of belonging. She named for herself her narrative and experience of Church as a place of restoration and solace, and God as ever-present and concerned about her struggles and well-being. This was an extraordinarily potent tool that we could make use of in therapy. Second, Colleen and I also expanded the narrative of what was happening in our therapeutic relationship. Our exploration that day led to a richer story of what we were doing together and the scope of what therapy meant. In some ways it brought together spheres of Colleen's experience that individually had the potential to help her, but that combined were exponentially more powerful.

Questions and Activities for Discussion and Further Reflection

1. Consider writing your own spiritual autobiography. You might do this as a journaling exercise or as something more formal. As with any personal and family history, go back a couple of generations. Were you raised in a spiritual tradition—even if only nominally? If so, which? What did you learn about it and the story it tells about the meaning of life and our existence? Was this typical of others from your tradition or not? How so?
2. What experiences have you had with different religious and spiritual traditions? Did you grow up in a place where most people were like you? Different from you? What was that like, and how do you feel it shaped you?
3. When you think of religious and spiritual differences, what feelings do they evoke in you? Curiosity? Discomfort? Ambivalence? What do you believe makes this so for you? How do you think it might impact your practice as a social worker?
4. If you were working with Colleen or another client like her, how do you sense it would have felt for you to ask about her spirituality and its place in her life? Consider role-playing a similar scenario with a peer and getting input from the class.
5. Go and learn about a spiritual or religious tradition that is different from your own and about which you do not know much. Talk to a spiritual leader of that tradition. Attend a service or other ritual. What does the tradition say about ultimate meaning? What might it be important for a social worker working with a member of that tradition to know?
6. Engage in a class discussion about the ways in which religious and spiritual differences appear in the news and social commentary today. Tune into and discuss the deeper social narrative you hear being told. What are the implications of this for us as social workers and our commitment to social justice?

7. Did any of the examples or stories in this chapter stand out to you in particular? If so, which ones? What in particular struck you about that narrative? Does it suggest anything to you about your own story or that of your clients?
8. Articulate for yourself your understanding of the most important factors for a social worker to keep in mind when trying to attend to spiritual narrative in our work with clients.

References

Albertsen, E. J., O'Connor, L. E., & Berry, J. W. (2006). Religion and interpersonal guilt: Variations across ethnicity and spirituality. *Mental Health, Religion & Culture, 9*(1), 67–84.

Altmaier, E. M. (2013). Through a glass darkly: Personal reflections on the role of meaning in response to trauma. *Counselling Psychology Quarterly, 26*(1), 106–113. https://doi.org/10.1080/09515070.2012.728760

Barker, S. L., & Floersch, J. E. (2010). Practitioners' understandings of spirituality: Implications for social work education. *Journal of Social Work Education, 46*(3), 357–370.

Bingaman, K. A. (2003). *Freud and faith: Living in the tension*. Albany, NY: State University of New York Press.

Bruner, J. (1990). *Acts of meaning*. Cambridge, MA: Harvard University Press.

Bruner, J. (1991). The narrative construction of reality. *Critical Inquiry, 18*(1), 1–21.

Canda, E. R., & Furman, L. D. (2009). *Spiritual diversity in social work practice: The heart of helping* (2nd ed.). New York: Oxford University Press.

Carlson, T. D., & Erickson, M. J. (2000). Re-authoring spiritual narratives: God in person's relational identity stories. *Journal of Systemic Therapies, 19*(2), 65–83.

Council on Social Work Education. (2015). *2015 educational policy and accreditation standards for baccalaureate and master's social work programs*. Alexandria, VA: Council on Social Work Education.

Cunningham, M. (2011). *Integrating spirituality in clinical social work practice: Walking the labyrinth*. New York: Pearson.

Figley, C. R. (1995). Compassion fatigue as secondary traumatic stress disorder: An overview. In C. R. Figley (Ed.), *Compassion fatigue: Coping with secondary traumatic stress disorder in those who treat the traumatized* (pp. 1–20). New York: Brunner-Routeldge.

Gay, P. (2006). *Freud: A life for our time*. New York: W.W. Norton.

Gockel, A. (2013). Telling the ultimate tale: The merits of narrative research in the psychology of religion. *Qualitative Research in Psychology, 10*(2), 189–203. https://doi.org/10.1080/14780887.2011.616622

Gurney, A. G., & Rogers, S. A. (2007). Object relations and spirituality: Revisiting a clinical dialogue. *Journal of Clinical Psychology, 63*(10), 961–977.

Hall, T. W. (2004). Christian spirituality and mental health: A relational spirituality framework for empirical research. *Journal of Psychology and Christianity, 23*, 66–81.

Hall, T. W. (2007). Psychoanalysis, attachment, and spirituality part I: The emergence of two relational traditions. *Journal of Psychology and Theology, 35*(1), 14–28.

Hodge, D. R. (2015). *Spiritual assessment in social work and mental health practice*. New York: Columbia University Press.

Hodge, D. R., & Horvath, V. E. (2011). Spiritual needs in health care settings: A qualitative metasynthesis of clients' perspectives. *Social Work, 56*(4), 306–316.

Lietz, C. A., & Hodge, D. R. (2013). Incorporating spirituality into substance abuse counseling: Examining the perspectives of service recipients and providers. *Journal of Social Service Research, 39*, 498–510.

MacIntyre, A. (1985). *After virtue: A study in moral theory* (2nd ed.). London, UK: Duckworth.

Martis, L., & Westhues, A. (2015). Religion, spirituality, or existentiality in bad news interactions: The perspectives and practices of physicians in India. *Journal of Religion and Health, 54*(4), 1387–1402. https://doi.org/10.1007/s10943-014-9959-3

McCann, I. L., & Pearlman, L. A. (1990). Vicarious traumatization: A framework for understanding the psychological effects of working with victims. *Journal of Traumatic Stress, 3*(1), 131–149.

McCullough, M. E., Pargament, K. I., & Thoresen, C. E. (2000). *Forgiveness: Theory, research, and practice*. New York: Guilford.

National Association of Social Workers. (2008). *The NASW code of ethics*. Washington, DC: NASW Press.

Naturale, A. (2007). Secondary traumatic stress in social workers responding to disasters: Reports from the field. *Clinical Social Work Journal, 35*, 173–181.

Northcut, T. B. (2000). Constructing a place for religion and spirituality in psychodynamic practice. *Clinical Social Work Journal, 28*(2), 155–169. https://doi.org/10.1023/A:1005102200804

Northcut, T. B. (2004). Pedagogy in diversity: Teaching religion & spirituality in the clinical social work classroom. *Smith College Studies in Social Work, 74*(2), 349–358. https://doi.org/10.1080/00377310409517720

Olson, T., Tisdale, T. C., Davis, E. B., Park, E. A., Nam, J., Moriarty, G. L., … Hays, L. W. (2016). God image narrative therapy: A mixed-methods investigation of a controlled group-based spiritual intervention. *Spirituality in Clinical Practice, 3*(2), 77–91. https://doi.org/10.1037/scp0000096

Oxhandler, H. K., & Pargament, K. I. (2014). Social work practitioners' integration of clients' religion and spirituality in practice: A literature review. *Social Work, 59*(3), 271–279.

Oxhandler, H. K., Parrish, D. E., Torres, L. R., & Achenbaum, W. A. (2015). The integration of clients' religion and spirituality in social work practice: A national survey. *Social Work, 60*(3), 228–237. https://doi.org/10.1093/sw/swv018

Pargament, K. I. (1997). *The psychology of religion and coping*. New York: Guilford Press.

Pargament, K. I. (2007). *Spiritually integrated psychotherapy: Understanding and addressing the sacred*. New York: The Guilford Press.

Pargament, K. I., Magyar-Russell, G. M., & Murray-Swank, N. A. (2005). The sacred and the search for significance: Religion as a unique process. *Journal of Social Issues, 61*(4), 665–687. https://doi.org/10.1111/j.1540-4560.2005.00426.x

Pearlman, L. A., & Saakvitne, K. W. (1995). Treating therapists with vicarious traumatization and secondary traumatic stress disorders. In C. R. Figley (Ed.), *Compassion fatigue: Coping with secondary traumatic stress disorder in those who treat the traumatized* (pp. 150–177). New York: Brunner-Routledge.

Pew Forum on Religion and Public Life. (2012, October 9). "Nones" on the rise. Retrieved from http://www.pewforum.org/2012/10/09/nones-on-the-rise/

Pew Research Center. (2014). The spiritual but not religious. Retrieved from http://www.pewforum.org/religious-landscape-study/religious-denomination/spiritual-but-not-religious/-demographic-information.

Rizzuto, A. (1974). Object relations and the formation of the image of god. *British Journal of Medical Psychology, 47*, 83–99.

Rizzuto, A. (1979). *The birth of the living god: A psychoanalytic study*. Chicago: University of Chicago Press.

Senreich, E. (2013). An inclusive definition of spirituality for social work education and practice. *Journal of Social Work Education, 49*(4), 548–563.

Stanley, M. A., Bush, A. L., Camp, M. E., Jameson, J. P., Phillips, L. L., Barber, C. R., … Cully, J. A. (2011). Older adults' preferences for religion/spirituality in treatment for anxiety and depression. *Aging & Mental Health, 15*(3), 334–343.

Tosone, C., McTighe, J. P., & Bauwens, J. (2015). Shared traumatic stress among social workers in the aftermath of Hurricane Katrina. *British Journal of Social Work, 45*(4), 1313–1329. https://doi.org/10.1093/bjsw/bct194

Tosone, C., McTighe, J. P., Bauwens, J., & Naturale, A. (2011). Shared traumatic stress and the long-term impact of 9/11 on Manhattan clinicians. *Journal of Traumatic Stress, 24*(5), 546–552. https://doi.org/10.1002/jts.20686

Tuval-Mashiach, R., & Dekel, R. (2014). Religious meaning-making at the community level: The forced relocation from the Gaza strip. *Psychology of Religion and Spirituality, 6*(1), 64–71. https://doi.org/10.1037/a0033917

Volkan, V. (1988). *The need to have enemies and allies: From clinical practice to international relationships*. New York: Jason Aronson.

White, M. (2007). *Maps of narrative practice*. New York: W.W. Norton.

White, M., & Epston, D. (1990). *Narrative means to therapeutic ends*. New York: W.W. Norton.

Wong, Y.-L. R., & Vinsky, J. (2009). Speaking from the margins: A critical reflection on the 'spiritual-but-not-religious' discourse in social work. *British Journal of Social Work, 39*(7), 1343–1359. https://doi.org/10.1093/bjsw/bcn032

Zinnbauer, B. J., Pargament, K. I., Cole, B., Rye, M. S., Butter, E. M., Belavich, T. G., … Kadar, J. L. (1997). Religion and spirituality: Unfuzzying the fuzzy. *Journal for the Scientific Study of Religion, 36*(4), 549–564.

Chapter 5
Sexual Stories: Narratives of Sexual Identity, Gender, and Sexual Development

Guiding Questions

What does narrative theory have to tell us about sexuality and its implications for clinical practice?

What do we mean by sexual identity and development and how can narrative help us understand and engage it as social workers?

In what ways does sexuality inform the developing sense of self of the individual in the social environment?

What are the dominant sexual narratives that are being told in the social and cultural world? How do these shape our own experience of sexuality as well as that of the clients with whom we work?

How may narrative help us to attend to issues of sexuality and sexual identity in the clinical encounter with our clients?

There is perhaps no dimension of our human experience that is simultaneously so shrouded in mystery, yet capable of sparking such visceral reactions as sexuality. The word itself conjures a whole host of associations: thoughts, emotions, memories, and bodily sensations. Perhaps that is because sexuality touches every part of our being in some way. Be in touch, for a moment, with everything that comes to you when you contemplate the word *sexuality*. For many of us, it is easiest and even automatic to focus on the first part of that word—sex. Yet I suggest that sexuality is about far more than genitals and how people choose to use them. Though you may not have thought about it in this way, I invite you to consider that sexuality is about the very life force that is at the heart of what it means to be human. Sexuality is the fundamental energy that fuels our capacity for love, connection, and intimacy. This is true even of platonic friendship. It lies at the root of a parent's love for his or her child, not only how that child was brought into being. It is the source of our ability to go beyond ourselves in the context of things like altruism and philanthropy, extending concern even to the stranger. For those of us who are social workers or clinicians of any discipline, I would argue that sexuality lies at the heart of the positive helping relationship we develop with our clients.

I will admit that there have been times when I have said these kinds of things in a classroom or a workshop and have encountered responses that ranged from confused to uncomfortable. How is sexuality related to my non-romantic friendships? How could sexuality have anything to do with a healthy love between parent and child, let alone with the feelings of concern I have toward humanity as a whole? And, as practitioners grounded responsibly in our Code of Ethics, what could sexuality possibly have to do with my relationship to my clients? I would suggest that this is because we have been conditioned to think about sexuality in particularly limiting ways. And that brings us back, once again, to the theory of social construction.

Recall that social construction looks at the way our human knowing and experiencing are conditioned on the social and cultural influences that we encounter in the world in which we live. The meaning of things like sexuality is informed and shaped by those social and cultural factors. This has a number of ramifications for the present discussion. For one thing, human beings take comfort in our ability to categorize experience in ways that are familiar and even predictable.

The French philosopher Michel Foucault (1978, 1979) critiqued the way we commonly give our assent to this kind of categorization of humanity and human experience without reflection, affording it the assumption of truth and validity. To some extent, we have a special appreciation for binary, if not to say polarized categories, some of which we conceive of along a spectrum (Gergen, 2015). We set in opposition to each other notions such as healthy and unhealthy, normal and abnormal, and innocence and guilt. Note that in these kinds of conceptual sets there is often an association to one of them as inherently good or at least preferable. Thus, health, normalcy, and innocence are commonly seen as better than their alternatives.

In the area of sexuality, at least in the West, we have similarly constructed the categories of male and female, masculine and feminine, and heterosexual and homosexual that polarize these dimensions of human experience (Gergen, 2015). As you read this, you might well find yourself thinking, "Well, wait a minute. What about people who identify as transgender? And we are not exclusively masculine or feminine. We all have aspects of both, right? What about people who identify as bisexual or even asexual?" Of course, as you pose these questions you are quite right. However, think about the way all of these qualifiers or more subtle nuances in our way of naming experience have evolved as social and cultural critiques of more fixed and dominant models. Contemplate the ways in which they are all the subject of ongoing social, cultural, and political debate.

In this chapter we consider narratives of human sexuality including constructs such as sexual identity, gender, and sexual development and functioning throughout the life span. We reflect on a variety of dimensions that may be pertinent for an understanding of the delicate complexity of the sexual narrative of the persons with whom we work—and our own as well—in addition to the meaning of all this for the therapeutic encounter and relationship. Sexuality and our sexual story have a way of being elusive, resistant to reduction, and difficult to contain. The sexual story has a way of awakening internal responses that may feel unfamiliar, and for some even threatening, evoking a particular set of defenses. This is especially true if sexuality is an area of life and the self in which someone has felt particularly wounded.

Come back for a moment to Foucault (1978, 1979) and his critique of an unreflective acceptance of the categories that a social and cultural power structure would offer as a container for our experience. You may recall from Chapt. 1 Bruner's (1991) discussion of the recursive relationship between narrative and culture—each in turn giving shape to the other. Recall too, that Bruner highlights the way in which culture establishes the range of interpretive options at our disposal as we attempt to make meaning of our experience. An expansion of that canon or framework of meanings requires a shift in the cultural discourse. For example, think of recent vigorous sociopolitical and cultural debates about gay marriage, transgender rights, and laws about which public restrooms individuals are allowed to use. I propose that in this chapter we engage in critical reflection on narratives of sexuality on individual as well as social and cultural levels, and the complex relationship between these stories. My hope is that this will lead us to a richer understanding of ourselves, our clients, and the therapeutic relationship we hope to establish with them.

So let's begin at the beginning. At some point at the start of your life, either while you were still in the womb via sonogram or at the very moment of your birth itself, someone almost certainly declared "It's a boy!" or "It's a girl!" and a narrative about a fundamental aspect of your personhood, complete with all its ambiguities, was begun. This narrative, based initially on an observation of your genitals, brought with it a host of assumptions about virtually every aspect of your life. Think about it. Everything from the clothes you would wear to the toys you would play with, and perhaps even the color of your room, was suggested by the presence of a penis or a vagina. If it so happened that you were born with ambiguous genitalia, this was certainly not overlooked and was likely met with some level of concern and subsequent testing. If your family chose to push back against gender-based stereotypes, the effort to do so still implies an acknowledgement of the cultural traditions and expectations they chose to defy. Later fantasies and associations about who you would become, what your interests or hobbies might be, what kind of career you might have, and so much more about you would be evoked by this mix of nature and nurture, biology, and cultural formation that is perhaps as indecipherable as it is inescapable.

Over the course of the life span, you have been exposed to countless messages about your body and your sexuality. Some of these have been very explicit and were felt to be welcome or not, or maybe a combination of both. Others have been so deeply imbedded in layers of cultural assumptions that they may be difficult even to recognize let alone call into question. They are like the air we breathe. Whether explicit or implicit, all of these images are mediated to us by the vehicles of our culture: the media, family, religion, social world, workplace, etc.

In the clinical context, this dimension of some clients' experience is going to be of far greater meaning and consequence than it is for others. However, even a cursory assessment of a client's sexual story and the history of their sexual development and sense of self can be useful in helping establish a context for such a foundational part of a client's life. A more in-depth exploration can be conducted when that is deemed to be important. Throughout the course of this chapter, we look at different aspects of the sexual story and how we might attend to them with our clients. This exploration of the sexual narrative is, of course, always to be undertaken in a context that is as supportive and free of judgment as possible.

So how do we set that kind of context or frame for our practice? Go back to the fundamental principles that guide all of our work and the establishment of the therapeutic relationship. We, as clinicians, need to be as well prepared and finely tuned as we can in order to best help our clients. This means knowing ourselves as well as possible and committing ourselves to the same process of ongoing growth and development in which we accompany our clients. In keeping with this, it is in our clients' best interest, and our own as well, if we have explored, understood, embraced, and even healed if necessary and as much as possible our own sexuality and sexual story.

Many years ago, I worked in an agency that had a fairly large training program for students. We would supervise interns who came from a variety of academic programs in social work, psychology, and counseling. Early in the course of her internship for her graduate program in counseling, Monica began working with a young woman who had presented for treatment to deal with the consequences of a sexual assault that she had experienced. These were the client's own words. She wrote them on one of the intake forms next to the question that asked her to describe briefly why she was coming for services. According to my colleague who was supervising her, Monica prepared a competent though not terribly rich intake evaluation and began to work with her client.

After several weekly sessions between Monica and the client, the supervisor noticed through progress notes and supervisory discussions that the topic of the sexual assault had not been touched. Instead, Monica would ask the client about the events of the week and other matters which, even if worthwhile, were not in line with the stated reason she was coming to therapy. So the supervisor addressed the issue with Monica in their weekly meeting. Had she discussed the sexual assault, the details of which were still unclear, with the client? Monica responded to the question with a mix of confusion and dismay. No, of course not, she replied. How could she possibly bring up something like that in the session? If the client chose to address it, she would listen. But she could never ask her about such a thing. That would be terribly intrusive. The supervisor reminded Monica that dealing with the sexual assault was the reason the client came to therapy. She had written it on the paperwork. Still, Monica insisted that she could not ask a client about the sexual assault she had experienced or even her sexuality in general. These issues were too deeply personal and even painful. Out of concern for the well-being of the client, she was soon transferred to another clinician.

Ask yourself how you would feel in Monica's shoes. Would you have been comfortable enough to ask the client about this part of her story? If the trauma the client needed to process had not touched on the area of her sexuality, would Monica have felt more confident addressing it? Perhaps. Though I do not know what specifically led to Monica's hesitation with this client, I would suggest that it is related to some aspect of her own narrative about sexuality, sexual assault, and what it means for something to be "too personal" for discussion, even in the context of therapy. I also believe that there are some important lessons to be learned here.

As in many other ways in the clinical encounter, clients will often take their cue from us regarding what they can talk about and how safe they can feel in the therapeutic space. One might wonder why, after having written what she did on the initial paper work, the client did not bring up the sexual assault in session. It's a good question. Perhaps the client wasn't ready to talk about this part of her narrative, even if she knew it was important. But perhaps the client mustered all of her courage to write it down, and was waiting for the therapist to follow up and signal that it was safe to talk about. Perhaps the client needed to know that the therapist could handle this part of her story. This is a moment when we stand at the intersection of our own narrative and that of our client. Our own countertransferential reactions (Counselman, 2014; White & Denborough, 2011) emerge from this narrative matrix and may, unwittingly, become an obstacle to working effectively with the client.

In my experience, this is quite common. We should of course never push a client to discuss an issue beyond what they can handle safely. They may at times feel quite uncomfortable in their therapeutic work as they explore difficult aspects of their story, but we don't want them to feel unsafe. In my own practice, this has often meant knowing when enough is enough—allowing a client to back away from a topic when it became too much for them to handle. This kind of moment invites us to return to work on containment and self-regulation. Similarly, as we discussed in Chap. 3, when a client is tempted to spill over or share, clinical wisdom tells us gently to help the client slow down so that they don't feel reactively unsafe afterwards. As with other difficult topics, I suggest that it is up to us to model safety, confidence, and comfort with clients by our ability to raise sensitive, even painful, topics. Especially if the issue raises fear or anxiety for the client, they need to know that we can handle it.

The idea of exploring sexuality and matters of sex can be intimidating for many clinicians, even experienced ones. For all kinds of reasons they may, like Monica, find the topic too delicate, complicated, or even private. However, I would encourage you to remember a couple of things. Unless you are a trained sex therapist, you are not expected to be an expert in all things sexual. In fact, you might have your own fair share of questions about sex and sexuality. However, my experience has been that clients' narratives of their sexuality rarely demand that specific a level of expertise. At the same time, the client who comes to us for treatment does not imagine that they are going to engage in cocktail party chitchat in which discussion of deeply personal matters would be taboo. They are coming to us for a reason—because we are professionals. Generally speaking, they want to talk about the things that most concern them, and they are relying on us not only for a body of information, which we can always keep acquiring, but also for a professional stance that communicates our preparedness to listen to them and care for them sensitively. This means being in touch with and working through our own issues and biases around sex and sexuality.

Consider then a study that was done by Logie, Bogo, and Katz (2015) in which they administered an objective structured clinical exam to social work students and recent graduates. The students conducted a 15-min interview with an African-Canadian actor playing a client who disclosed to the social worker some conflicted feelings about her same-sex attraction, not at all an uncommon scenario. In processing this exercise, a number of important findings emerged from the beginning therapists' reactions. These students and new social workers identified feelings of anxiety and other manifestations of discomfort when the client "came out." They noted an increase in self-consciousness and questioned their own preparedness to handle this part of the client's story.

On a perhaps more subtle, but deeply important level, a number of the subjects were aware of their own surprise when the client disclosed her sexual orientation, and their presumption of the client's heterosexuality. The authors highlight this as evidence of the widespread heterosexism that exists in our society and the resultant pressure that some diverse clients feel to hide their sexual identity even from providers, or to question whether it will be accepted.

All this implies some important things for us. Not only is it essential for us to know our own sexual narrative and ourselves well enough to recognize the issues we find challenging, but we also have to work purposefully at developing our skills and managing our own feelings and reactions in order to provide our clients with the kind of treatment they need and deserve. In keeping with this, we need to know how our own attitudes and beliefs have been shaped by our immersion in the social and cultural surround of our experience.

Like most social workers I would wager, the students and new social workers in this study were not consciously narrow minded or willfully biased. In fact, the subjects held consciously positive attitudes toward members of the LGBT community. But when put in a practice situation in which they were asked to sit with this important aspect of the sexual story of a client, they came face to face with some of their own limitations of skill and the more negative beliefs and stereotypes they had internalized from the culture at large (Logie et al., 2015).

This leads us to a consideration of an important theoretical perspective rooted in social constructionism that can serve as an interpretive framework for this discussion. Beginning in the early 1970s the theory of sexual scripting emerged as a means of understanding the socially constructed nature of sexuality and sexual behavior (Gagnon & Simon, 1973; Simon & Gagnon, 2003). According to this theory, the nature and meaning of sexuality and sexual experience are about far more than the body. They are inextricably tied to the social and historical situation in which they are lived (Simon & Gagnon, 2003). From our understanding of gender and our relationship to our own and others' bodies, to both the public and private enactments of our sexuality, sexual scripts condition the cultural, interpersonal, and intrapersonal meanings of sexuality (Masters, Casey, Wells, & Morrison, 2013).

What does that mean? For starters, think about the way in which an understanding of sex and sexuality has evolved over the course of time and across different cultures. What, for example, does it mean to be beautiful? Or feminine, masculine, or desirable? Whose sexuality and sexual behavior are considered "normal" or "abnormal, and by whom? What social consequences are granted or imposed as a result of being "normal" or "abnormal"? What sexual behaviors are considered healthy and unhealthy? Moral and immoral? What does it mean to be a man? A woman? Even before we reach the stage of adolescence and experience the awakening of our own genital sexual desires, we are implicitly aware of many of the culturally reinforced messages about sexuality that surround us (Gagnon, Rosen, & Leiblum, 1982). In fact, these scripts are so deeply embedded in our sense of self and the world that they are often not even noticed until they break down or are challenged in some way (Gagnon et al., 1982).

Mitchell et al. (2011) outlined three sexual scripts that emerged as operating in their research. They are the biomedical, the relational, and the erotic. The biomedical script focuses on the genital experience of sex with its expected culmination in orgasm. The relational script emphasizes the importance of intimacy and emotional connection in the sexual relationship. The erotic script highlights the desire for excitement and the search for new kinds of sexual experience. One can see how these three dimensions of the relationship to sex and sexuality connect with and emerge from diverse messages about the meaning of the body and of the pursuit of sexual engagement. Depending on which script or scripts are dominant for us, we may evaluate ourselves, our bodies, and our sexual experience, or lack thereof, quite differently.

These socially constructed messages do of course evolve. Recall Bruner's (1991) observation that we are shaped by culture and society and in turn have a hand in shaping them. This is the process by which culturally dominant scripts change over time. The same may be said about our sense of sex and sexuality. Masters et al. (2013), for example, studied young heterosexual men and women to understand how their gender-related scripts impacted their experience of relationships. Even though the subjects' way of thinking about masculine and feminine behavior was in line with the dominant socially constructed understandings of these constructs, the authors found that these young people had a variety of ways of relating to them in their actual lives. Some of the subjects *conformed* to the dominant cultural script in their own personal behavior. Others engaged in *exception finding* in which they allowed themselves to deviate from the cultural gender script in some way while still giving their assent to it. Finally, others sought to *transform* the cultural script by enacting an alternative personal script in their own life and behavior and promoting that alternative as equally or more valid.

The examples of these ways of relating to cultural scripts are numerous and far-reaching. One has only to think about the social constructions that have governed issues like women in the workplace. Think about the fact that there was a time, not very long ago, when women's roles were predominantly confined to the home. When women were found in the workplace, the cultural expectation was that they were generally limited to certain kinds of jobs and functions, typically of a supportive nature (e.g., secretaries). Conversely, men have been culturally expected to be the "bread winner," and to be chiefly responsible for the financial support of the family. I have worked with men who struggled with the fact that their wives or girlfriends made more money than they did. Even when they knew intellectually that there was "nothing wrong with that" they felt that it challenged the role they felt they were expected to fulfill.

I recall that, when I was in social work school, I went with my supervisor for lunch one day in the hospital cafeteria. After we had gotten our food, she saw a table of other social workers and we went to join them. Out of the ten or so people at the table, I was the only man, and the only student. Being an intern and not knowing any of them very well, I remained largely quiet and listened. At some point the conversation turned to the topic of social work as a field and the relatively low pay that social workers could expect to earn. One woman said, and the others generally agreed, "The only reason I can afford to be a social worker is that my husband makes a lot of money." As a student—and the only man present—I have to admit that it left me to wonder what this meant for *my* future in social work. It also struck me as a complex statement about gender-based expectations and cultural scripts related to work, money, and responsibility.

Even in our contemporary context in which the presence of both men and women in the workplace is generally normative (though certain patterns of gender domination in some fields still exist), we continue to be engaged in cultural debates about issues like equal pay for equal work. The nature of the scripts that inform our way of seeing the world tends to hang on and change only slowly. Current social and cultural dialogues about issues such as the experience of transgendered persons, gay marriage, and the civil and legal rights of same-sex couples are signs of an ongoing, sometimes heated, and often politically polarized evolution of the social meaning of sex and sexuality.

Lest all of this seem very abstract and far removed from the realities of daily living, let's not lose sight of the way in which these kinds of constructs manifest themselves in and impact our lives and those of our clients. From a broad developmental point of view, it can be helpful to understand the way in which maleness and femaleness, and masculinity and femininity, were modeled for us and came to be part of our foundational sexual narrative. What did we see and take in about these attributes? For some of us, the messages we received were quite fixed and expectations were clear. Boys are like this. Girls are like that. These expectations likely had much to do with external factors such as how we dressed, walked, and talked, as well as the interests and activities we engaged in and that were endorsed as being appropriate or not. But they also had a great deal to do with more internal dispositions like how we were taught to relate to our emotions and the range of feelings that was deemed appropriate for us to express (Brown, Craig, & Halberstadt, 2015; van der Pol et al., 2015; Zaman & Fivush, 2013).

It has been my experience that these issues come up routinely in treatment. Though it may seem in some ways like a cliché, a particular expression of it comes when we work with couples who may be in conflict because they are talking past each other in some way. Mark and Stephanie, for example, came to treatment when they found themselves having an increasingly hard time managing the frequency and intensity of their arguments at home. Mark worked long hours at a corporate job and Stephanie was a stay-at-home mom. The parents of three young children, they found themselves busy throughout the day and exhausted by the evening. With little time together, their communication became more perfunctory and focused on the business of the household. As their level of conflict grew, they could feel the distance growing between them. Things came to a head one night when they found themselves discussing whether they would be better off separating. It was a sobering talk. They both realized that neither of them wanted a divorce, but they knew that things couldn't continue as they were either.

As we began to explore the roots of their concerns, particular themes emerged in their individual narratives that led us to explore their stories of what it means to be a man or woman, a husband or wife. At the end of a long day, Stephanie was eager to find in Mark a listening and supportive ear—someone who could convey a sense of understanding about the many things she had juggled throughout the day. Instead, her narrative was that she was, for Mark, nothing more than the next thing he had to attend to in his day, an item to check off on his to-do list. She felt as if Mark was waiting only to ask, "So, what do you need me to do?" For his part, Mark reported that he understood that Stephanie juggled an enormous amount throughout the day. He wanted to be helpful and felt the best way to do this was through problem solving, planning, and taking whatever he could off her plate. He wanted to be a supportive husband but admitted that he grew increasingly resentful as he felt that none of his initiatives were acknowledged by Stephanie or made any difference. What more could she possibly want from him?

We began to explore both Mark and Stephanie's families of origin. What emerged were some striking parallels in the narratives of growing up in their respective homes and what they learned, even without realizing it, about their gender roles. Mark and Stephanie both grew up in very traditional, Caucasian, middle class homes with hardworking fathers and equally hard-working, stay-at-home mothers. Neither recalled seeing or hearing their parents talk much about life, work, raising children, or managing the details of busy lives. In fact, what they each saw was a fairly stark divide. While their mothers took care of all things related to the home and the kids, their fathers were quiet and somewhat distant. Even though they were present for most activities and family events, they rarely communicated much or expressed emotion. They occupied themselves mostly with work and some occasional hobbies. I encouraged both Mark and Stephanie to put into words the story that they took away from their childhood homes about these gender roles and what they wanted for their own lives. Each in their own way gave voice to a wish for something more: more engagement, more communication, and more sharing. But they struggled to say much more than that.

As we wondered about this together, both Mark and Stephanie found themselves increasingly in touch with some feelings that began to shift the narrative of what was happening in their own relationship. Each of them was telling themselves a story of what their wished-for "something more" would look like. The issue was that their stories weren't coming together. Though they did not want to replicate in their own marriage what they saw as the stereotypical behavior or scripts they had seen in their parents, they nonetheless realized that they were in fact enacting some very traditional socially constructed roles. With patient attention, Mark was able to hear that Stephanie was looking to establish an emotional connection with him at the end of the day, wanting him simply to hear her and take in all that she had to say. For her part, Stephanie was able to hear that Mark felt the weight of responsibility to be helpful and to take perceived burdens off Stephanie's shoulders. His, "What do you need me to do?" was intended to be an expression of solidarity and concern, not a dismissal. His sense of his role was to make things better, and this entailed not just listening, but doing—a very typical Western male notion. For his part, Mark came to understand that Stephanie did not in fact need or want him to *do* any more. Her venting about the day was a way of seeking connection and intimacy. Her sense of her role was to tend to relationships, and this entailed the mutual act of sharing and listening—a very typical Western female notion.

Consistent with Masters et al.'s (2013) findings, each of us is brought up in a world in which we are immersed in this complex set of assumptions and expectations about our sexuality. Similarly, our experience of our gender and the implications of our sexed body can be profoundly meaningful. In addition to reflecting on the story we inherited from our role models based on what we saw of their masculinity and/or femininity, we can also ask how the world around us received our own gender. Was our sexuality, in this sense, celebrated and affirmed? Was it regretted or denied? Was it perceived as threatened or threatening? So many people carry with them into their adulthood the legacy of feeling unwanted or unseen in their gendered self—a sense of being somehow not enough—not masculine enough or feminine enough, not conforming enough to the expectations of the world around us, or confused as to what those expectations were. These expectations were mediated to us not only by adults of the same sex, but often in significant ways by those of the opposite sex. Thus, the impact of fathers on the gendered experience of their daughters and mothers on their sons can be of enormous developmental significance (Barnett & Scaramella, 2013; Hess, Ittel, & Sisler, 2014; Lamb & Lewis, 2010).

Patricia was an adult survivor of incest by her father who had been in therapy for some time when she began to talk with her therapist about some new feelings she was experiencing toward her 13-year-old son. She had always experienced a particular closeness with her son, a unique bond that she enjoyed deeply. However, in the past several months, she told her therapist, she had become aware of feelings of aggression and resentment toward him. She did not know where these feelings came from, but Patricia found herself simultaneously drawn in and repulsed by them. She very much disliked these reactions toward her son, but experienced the feelings as almost irresistible. The therapist confirmed that there was no actual physical aggression or any other form of abuse happening in the home, and began to explore Patricia's feelings with her. As she reflected on the change that had taken place in her reactions, Patricia came to realize that things began to shift for her when she noticed her son going through puberty. Even at 13, Patricia could see changes beginning in her son's body, his size and shape, his odor, and beginnings of hair growing on his body. They represented for Patricia signs of the man her son was slowly becoming.

This was a key moment in her understanding of her story. With her therapist's help, Patricia was able to get in touch with a deeply painful part of her narrative. Beginning with her own father and extending to relationships with other men in her life, Patricia realized that she had few positive experiences of men that she could hold onto. Rather, her experience was that men were controlling and abusive, and almost always took advantage of women. Thus, Patricia came to fear that her son would grow to be like so many of the other men she had known. As a boy of 13, however, her son was still very much dependent on his mother, and the development of his body and his character both had a long way to go. As she got in touch with the shift that was taking place within her, Patricia resolved to work with her therapist on how not only to refrain from acting out against her son and his emerging masculinity, but also to help him grow to become the best man he could be. She realized that as a woman and his mother, she had an enormous impact on the development of her son. In this way, Patricia discovered a positive direction for the transformation of a piece of her narrative of sexuality—both masculine and feminine.

Clients from diverse racial backgrounds may experience another dimension of these culturally reinforced narratives of sexuality. A number of scholars have examined the way in which expectations of sexuality and sexual behavior are conditioned not only on gender but on race as well (Fasula, Carry, & Miller, 2014; Montemurro, 2017; Saketopoulou, 2011). This particular manifestation of intersectionality has led some to describe a sexual double standard to which some people may be subjected. These authors suggest that African-American women and other women of color, for example, may have to contend with a cultural story that paints them as hypersexual in contrast to women of other races, and as sexually assertive in the face of cultural expectations of men's sexual dominance and women's sexual passivity (Fasula et al., 2014; Montemurro, 2017). In these narratives, women and men run the risk of not being allowed to explore the meaning of their own sexuality, their sexual body, and their sexual choices, but of having their story conditioned for them on the basis of both gender and race. Within and across cultures, we use these stories to establish what we believe to be norms and expectations regarding things like sex drive and sexual prowess, number of sexual partners and frequency of sex, and even sexual orientation. These kinds of narratives of sexuality and sexual behavior, elaborated along the lines of racial group and gender, can become yet another way in which both women and men may be oppressed by stereotyped cultural scripts.

Narratives of Genital Sexuality

This leads us to the exploration of another key aspect of the sexual narrative, the story of our genital sexuality. As noted at the beginning of this chapter, perhaps the most common associations about sexuality pertain to our genitals and what we choose to do with them. And yet, our understanding of what it means to inhabit our sexual body can often lack depth. In point of fact, our experience of our genital sexuality is highly nuanced and brings with it a wider range of both internal and social responses and expectations.

Begin by asking yourself when you first became aware of yourself as genitally sexual. Perhaps even in early childhood you had experiences that called your attention to the ways in which male and female bodies were different from each other, as well as the fact that not all male or female bodies were exactly the same. These may have been quite benign events such as the birth of a sibling of a different gender or the family rituals of bath time. At some point you also became aware of the role of your genitals in the experience of your sexuality. Think about when this first occurred for you. For many people, this consciousness of their genital sexuality emerged in relationship to the changes of puberty.

For a large part of my career I have worked with late adolescents and young adults. In the course of conducting a comprehensive initial assessment I have found it important to understand in some depth these clients' stories of puberty and early adolescence. As perhaps the most profound recent developmental milestone in their young life, the experience of puberty has meaning not only on a biological level, but on social and intrapersonal levels as well. Over time, I have been struck by the ways in which this entirely expectable developmental transition has impacted clients' narratives of their sexuality and sense of self.

I will commonly ask clients to recall how old they were when they became aware that they were experiencing puberty and what experience they use to mark that. For females, this is often the onset of menses or the noticeable development of their breasts. For males, this has most commonly been associated with the growth of body hair, the onset of body odor, or the increased frequency of, sometimes inexplicable, erections. Adolescents typically have a sense of whether their development feels early or late or on an expected course, often determined by comparison to peers. Many times, particularly if they feel that some aspect of their development is early or late, this can bring with it a host of feelings of self-consciousness, embarrassment, pride, or even worry. A significant part of the adolescent narrative as a whole is concerned with their place in the social world and their ability to fit into the social fabric—the story they tell themselves about themselves, each other, and what is considered "normal." The experience of the development of their genital sexuality and the effort to grow into a comfortable sense of their body as sexual in this specific sense are no exceptions.

Beyond the physical developments associated with puberty and the ways these awaken us to changes in our sexuality, we also become aware of the experience of sexual arousal and sexual attraction. Adolescents may begin to engage in masturbation in a new way or for the first time may engage in sexual experimentation or activity with others, and may come to an increasing sense of their sexual orientation. The way in which they experience or anticipate that their sexuality will be received by the world around them has an enormous role to play in their developing sense of self. Take a moment to contemplate the impact of these events on the unfolding sexual narrative and to be in touch with the variety of social and cultural messages that may seek to contribute meaning to these new and often confusing experiences. Is my sexuality welcomed, affirmed, and celebrated? Or it is a source of shame, confusion, or other conflict for me or those around me (e.g., family, friends)? Do I feel that I am attractive to others and desirable? Do not lose sight of the socially constructed narrative of what is considered attractive. How has this impacted my participation, or lack thereof, in romantic relationships? What do I perceive or tell myself about others' sexuality? What do others, particularly the objects of my romantic interest, value in me? And how does that fit into the broader narrative of my self in the world? Am I seen for the wholeness of who I am? How does my physical sexuality play into this? Is it stereotyped or caricatured in some way?

Amy was a 19-year-old young woman who came to see me to deal with the mild depressive feelings she'd been struggling with for a few years. Though she was bright and could point to a variety of accomplishments in academics and sports, she lacked self-confidence. She had a supportive family and a network of friends, but was uncertain that she was genuinely liked. One particular aspect of her life to which she returned often was her relationship to her boyfriend of 2 years. They were the same age and had met in their senior year of high school. She spoke of the relationship in stable terms and recounted how much they loved each other. They had begun to be sexually active together within a couple of months of dating. Each was the other's first sexual partner.

I began to notice that when Amy spoke about her boyfriend she often talked about their sexual interactions and the kinds of sexual behaviors they engaged in. At times, Amy expressed some ambivalence about their sex life and its role in the relationship. There were certain sexual behaviors, for example, that she didn't enjoy but did anyway. When I explored other aspects of her relationship to her boyfriend, the topic returned before long to sex. At times, she felt that sex dominated their plans or their time together. Where could they go for sex? Would they be alone?

I asked Amy if she had talked with her boyfriend about this and communicated to him her wish that sex would not have such a dominant place in the relationship. Amy paused and looked at me with genuine confusion. "But if I didn't have sex with him why would he be with me?" I invited her to tell me more. She said that her boyfriend was a good guy but that if she didn't offer what he liked and wanted sexually he would just leave her and find someone else who would. Amy told me that it had never occurred to her that she might be desirable as a woman for other aspects of her personhood. From the beginning, she said, she became sexually active because she felt it was what was required if she wanted to have a relationship.

Therapy began to explore her sense of self more broadly and the role that sex and sexuality played in the narrative of herself in the world. We explored Amy's story about love and relationships—what they meant and what the role of sex was in them. As she grew in self-confidence, she found that she was increasingly able to make choices about relationships and sex on her own terms and assert her own wishes with her boyfriend. This story isn't at all uncommon, of course, for adolescents and even for adults of all genders and sexual orientations. It serves, however, to highlight the way sex and sexual behavior function as a part of an overall narrative of our sense of self and our sexuality in the social context.

If we reflect on the question of when we first sensed that others noticed us as genitally sexual and the nature and meaning of that experience, we must be deeply mindful of those who have been the victims of childhood sexual abuse and other forms of sexual assault. Making meaning of these experiences can be extremely challenging for those whose lives have been affected by them (Anderson & Hiersteiner, 2008; Draucker et al., 2011). The early imposition of genital sexual experience by abuse and assault can have enduring consequences for the developing narrative of the self (Saha, Chung, & Thorne, 2011). Krayer, Seddon, Robinson, and Gwilym (2015), for example, studied the adult narratives of 30 survivors of childhood sexual abuse and identified three views of the self that predominated. The *worthless self* was characterized by poor self-esteem, negative emotions, and self-destructive behaviors such as substance abuse and self-harm. These had a manifest impact on the quality of adult connections of the subjects, leading them in some cases to find themselves in subsequent abusive relationships with others. The *self as unknown* related both to gaps in actual memory associated with the abuse and to the ongoing unresolved question of who the survivor might have been or what their life might have been like had the abuse not occurred. This sense of the self as unknown also then became a barrier in adult relationships to feeling known by significant others or to letting others in. There is a particular kind of pain, I suggest, in this struggle inasmuch as the answer to such a nagging question is fundamentally unknowable and even illusory. Finally, the *potential/developing self* referred to subjects' sense that they had in fact made progress on the road to healing from the wounds of their abuse and toward discovering something positive about themselves.

Researchers have also highlighted the role narrative plays in children's effort to make meaning of and heal from the experience of childhood sexual abuse (Mossige, Jensen, Gulbrandsen, Reichelt, & Tjersland, 2005). The elaboration of a coherent narrative is an integral part of the working through of traumatic experiences of this nature (Kamya, 2012; Schauer, Neuner, & Elbert, 2011). This is in line with Bruner's (1990) view that narrative is particularly called upon when life events unfold in unexpected ways. In these instances, the creation of stories helps us restore a sense of narrative flow.

Grossman, Sorsoli, and Kia-Keating (2006) examined the narratives of 16 male survivors of childhood sexual abuse to understand how they made meaning of that experience. Three such strategies were identified. The first, *action*, involved the transformation of experience by trying to help others in need or to find some creative outlet (e.g., art, music, writing) to give expression to the meaning of their trauma. Second, participants used a *cognitive framework* to come to some understanding of their abuse. This involved a range of approaches including the effort to understand the perpetrator as well as the self, and to set their abuse in some sociocultural or philosophical context. Third, some of the men interviewed drew a sense of meaning from their *spirituality* whether that involved traditional religion or another path such as a 12-step program.

As clinicians, we must sometimes grapple with the fact that this effort at meaning making does not necessarily imply that clients' conclusions will appear to us to be realistic or even helpful. Peter was in his mid-30s when he came to therapy, by his report, for his anxiety and interpersonal struggles. During the intake he told me that he and his wife had been married for 13 years and that they had three children, two boys and a girl. He also disclosed that when he was about 10 years of age, he had been sexually abused by an adult male acquaintance of his father whom his parents had taken in and given a second bed in Peter's bedroom. According to Peter's recollection and understanding, his parents did not know the man very well, but he was a newly arrived immigrant from their country in Eastern Europe and was without a place to stay. As immigrants themselves, Peter's parents felt that it was their duty to help him out. Peter was uncomfortable with the stranger sleeping in his room, but out of respect said nothing to his parents.

After only a couple of weeks, Peter was awakened in the night by the man sitting on the bed next to him fondling Peter's genitals. Terrified, Peter pretended to be asleep, and after some time the man returned to his own bed. Peter told no one about what happened. The almost nightly routine of abuse that followed escalated past the point where Peter could feign sleep. The fondling of his genitals progressed to him being forced to fondle the abuser. Oral and anal sex soon became part of the cycle of abuse. In the morning, the man would behave as if nothing had occurred. He made casual conversation with Peter's parents at the breakfast table before dressing and heading off to his job at a local factory. To the best of Peter's recollection, the abuse lasted nearly 6 months, and ended only when the man moved into his own apartment. Through all of this Peter did not disclose the abuse to anyone. Even as an adult he was convinced that his parents would not have believed him. These things were not common in his culture, he insisted. In his whole life, he had only spoken about it on a handful of occasions and there were only a couple of people who knew of it, one of them being his wife.

In the process of exploring the experience of the abuse, it became clear that Peter suffered from some mild posttraumatic stress. There were still situations that Peter avoided. These included certain sexual positions and behaviors that reminded him of episodes of abuse. At times when something triggered a memory of the abuse, he could feel an increase in his anxiety. There were days, he reported, when he felt like he "checked out" mentally for up to a few minutes at a time. Peter's effort to make meaning of the experience, however, took him in a direction that he found even more challenging than these occasional symptoms.

From his early adolescence, Peter felt deeply conflicted about what he described as his same-sex attraction. A deeply religious man, he believed his urges and feelings to be inherently sinful and no part of God's plan for him. In keeping with what he understood to be God's will he dated two girls in his teens, eventually marrying the second of these, his wife. He had a couple of superficial same-sex encounters prior to marriage, but nothing since. His attraction to men had not changed over the years, but Peter continually prayed that they would and that he would be free of them. He spoke of his wife as a good woman whom he loved and who was attractive. In an effort to live what he deemed to be a normal life, he had sex with her periodically. He reported that he did not believe she was aware of his same-sex attraction, but rather attributed their infrequent sex to Peter having a minimal sexual appetite. She did not push him for more.

In Peter's narrative, his same-sex attraction was the direct result of having been abused by a man. This was his way of making meaning of sexual feelings he had no other way of accommodating in his view of God, himself, and the world. As a logical extension of this narrative thread, Peter assumed that all gay men had been sexually abused as children. Any effort to suggest, even gently, that this might not be the case—that there were gay men who had not been abused and, for that matter, survivors of abuse who were not gay—was met with polite but unyielding opposition. This simply couldn't be the case from Peter's point of view. Even at the expense of his happiness and peace of mind, the irrevocable connection he saw between his deeply painful experience of childhood sexual trauma and his adult sexual feelings allowed Peter to assign his attraction to men the status of a symptom. The more he worked at healing his trauma, he told himself, and the more he prayed for healing from his past, the more likely he believed his attractions would resolve themselves and he would be free to live what he saw as the life of a normal man. What's more, Peter suspected that to the extent he was not freed of these feelings it might be due to his own immorality and unworthiness. It is not surprising that this deep conflict, born of the mix of a terrifying story of abuse and the inability to embrace his adult sexuality, took a toll on Peter emotionally and interpersonally. It gave rise to the significant anxiety he struggled to manage on a daily basis. It made his effort to connect on a genuine level with both men and women fraught with tension and uncertainty. Peter felt alone and, not surprisingly, somewhat persecuted by God and by life.

Though the narrative path that Peter took was unique to him in many ways, the conflict he experienced in his sexuality has much to say to anyone who has struggled to be at ease with that part of their identity. Peter is a survivor of childhood sexual abuse, and that brings with it a host of potential complications all on its own. For others, however, the story line is quite different. As social workers, we are given the privilege of creating a space in which we can receive the stories of people who feel often quite vulnerable in one way or another, and advocate for them as needed.

Intimacy and Power

Take a moment and ask yourself what have you learned about the relationship between intimacy and sexuality? Power and sexuality? As we've seen, we come by this learning both implicitly and explicitly. It is communicated to us through the narrative of our family and our immediate surrounding, as well as through the social and cultural context at large. So what have you learned? Is intimacy always connected to sexuality? Does sex always involve intimacy? Whether from personal experience, friends, or some good television or movie drama, you have probably learned something about the complex social and sexual phenomenon referred to today as "friends with benefits"—the notion of friends engaging in sex for fun and with no emotional ties or expectations. What could go wrong? In spite of those initial intentions, someone often winds up feeling unexpectedly emotionally attached, and even hurt. When sex is seen simply as a leisure activity, the subtle meanings of sex and the vulnerability that comes with it may be overlooked.

For others, sex and sexuality have come to be associated with a story of threat and vulnerability. This may be true of a survivor not only of childhood abuse but also of rape or any other form of sexual assault. Sometimes this story evolves such that clients go out of their way to make themselves less attractive in some fashion (e.g., changes in weight, dress, grooming, etc.), believing that if they make themselves less attractive it will afford them an additional measure of protection. Women and members of sexual minority groups especially have often experienced their sexuality as a source of threat or vulnerability in the workplace, knowing that their gender, gender identity, or sexual orientation created a double standard that could lead to anything from outright harassment to perhaps more subtle expressions like the limiting of opportunities or unequal compensation for their work. For those who also identify with racial or other minority statuses, the intersection of these factors has led to environments that may be even more hostile (Fasula et al., 2014; Montemurro, 2017).

From a different point of view, it is also true that some engage in sex as a way of avoiding intimacy and a deeper emotional connection. For many people, it is far easier to take off their clothes and be physically naked with another, even someone they barely know, than it is to risk the emotional nakedness of revealing their heart and mind. I have sat with clients who sought one uncharted sexual frontier after another, hoping that it would bring them the experience of connection they simultaneously desired and feared, only to find that kind of intimacy beyond their reach. And I have known others whose instinct was to sexualize themselves and their encounters with others as a way of avoiding having to be truly known. In these instances, clients typically have a narrative that offers a view of intimacy as more frightening than sex, and the vulnerability it entails less tolerable.

One manifestation of that is the role of pornography, the proliferation of which has been so expansive in the age of the Internet. Seen by many men and women as a quick and accessible means of sexual excitement and release, it is in other ways a reduction of the complex meanings of sexuality to the sum of its parts—literally. Pornography relies in many ways on the anonymity that is required for viewers to focus solely on the erotic qualities of the body parts of their choice and to project, if they wish, their fantasy onto the bodies of others. Even pornography that purports to feature relationships, such as the amateur pornography of "real couples" and the "relationship-based" pornography often marketed more directly to women, is based, ironically, on the illusion of a staged intimacy between the people involved.

All of these examples are manifestations of particular social and cultural narratives that shape not only our individual lives but also how we interact with each other. Yet another aspect of this relates to the stories we tell ourselves about the relationship between sexuality and power. What is your sense of what the world says to you about the power or lack of power that is derived from your sexuality and the sexual nature of your being? Is it a power over someone else? Is that narrative empowering or disempowering? In certain ways, the social context is filled with messages about sex and sexuality as something so desirable that it may be wielded to get what we want. In other ways, many people feel profoundly disenfranchised in the world because of their sexuality. Those whose experience has told them that their gender and/or sexuality do not fit into the cultural master narrative of what is normal have had to cope with the invisibility and even rejection that come with being part of a minority (Hammack, Thompson, & Pilecki, 2009). Though it may be argued that some of that narrative has begun to shift, at least in some places in the culture, work on these issues is clearly not over.

To Be Sexually Active or Abstinent

Yet another dimension of narratives of sexuality is the meanings we ascribe to sexual activity itself, as well as to sexual functioning. Recall Amy about whom I wrote earlier in the chapter? You may remember that part of Amy's sexual narrative pertained to her assumption that unless she offered him sex, her boyfriend would not want to be with her. This had been an integral part of her decision to become sexually active in the first place. She had come to understand that this was what you do when you're in a relationship. She had not really entertained the question of whether or not she wanted to have sex yet, or if she felt ready for it.

In working with late adolescents and young adults, a question I typically ask when exploring sexuality during initial assessment is "Are you sexually active?" A common enough response to that question would be something along the lines of "What do you mean by sexually active?" to which I would reply somewhat playfully, "What do *you* mean by sexually active?" In point of fact, I have found the term can mean quite a variety of things. For some clients it connotes any kind of genital interaction with another person. For others, however, the definition is more limited, referring only to penile-vaginal intercourse, for example, depending on their sexual orientation. Other sexual behavior, even including oral and anal sex, might not "count." Regardless of whatever a "textbook" definition of the term *sexually active* might be, what matters here is what it means to the persons involved. In other words, their definition and the appraisal of their own behavior fit into a socially constructed narrative of what it means to be sexually active.

Other dimensions of this narrative include the sense of what might constitute the appropriate time and context for sex, with whom to have it and how often, and what the choice of sexual behavior says about the persons involved. Is sex something to be engaged in recreationally or out of curiosity? Is it meant to be experienced only in the context of a loving, committed relationship? Should sex be reserved for marriage only? Who is an appropriate vs. inappropriate person to have sex with? How long do you have to know a person before having sex with them? How young is too young to have sex? Is there a point when you've waited too long? Take stock of the thoughts and feelings you have in response to these questions and the ways in which your answers or perspectives are at once so personal and yet connected to the overall social narrative of which we are a part, a narrative that has shifted considerably over time. And make no mistake about the fact that people often have very strong opinions of themselves and others based on their answers to these questions and others like them. In complex social ways, decisions about sex and sexual activity cause some to be envied or admired and others to be reviled and shamed. Some of this occurs along traditional gender lines, at times assigning a reputation of great sexual prowess and success to one while labeling another a slut or some other pejorative term. Though often premature, adolescents often attribute to themselves and peers a somewhat artificial sense of maturity or the achievement of adulthood when they have begun to engage in sexual relationships.

The flip side of this discussion of what it means to be sexually active pertains to what it means both literally and socially to be a virgin. For some, especially some young people, virginity is a source of embarrassment while for others it is held as a mark of virtue. The desire to retain one's virgin status is often a part of the idiosyncratic definitions of what constitutes sexual activity (Carpenter, 2005).

As with the choice to be sexually active in whatever form, the choice to remain a virgin or to be sexually abstinent may be motivated by a number of personal and social factors. Cooke-Jackson, Orbe, Johnson, and Kauffman (2015) studied 65 undergraduate students (75% female, 25% male) who self-identified as virgins (defined as never having engaged in vaginal, oral, or anal sex) in order to understand the motivations for their abstinence. The first distinction observed was between conscious abstinence and involuntary abstinence. Members of the latter group attributed their lack of sex to causes such as lack of opportunity or not feeling sexually attractive and desired. Those who identified as consciously abstinent referred to a number of factors that contributed to their decision. Among these, religious or spiritual motivations made it important for some participants to wait for sex until marriage. Others reported that they were waiting for a committed relationship and to meet the right person with whom they would want to have sex. Still others recounted the fears they had related to having sex. These ranged from fears of pregnancy and sexually transmitted infections to the emotional risk of having a bad experience with someone who did not care about them.

During clinical assessment, in addition to ascertaining whether or not a person is sexually active and the age at which they first became sexually active, I try to understand what the experience meant to the person and how they feel looking back on it. For many people, the experience of losing their virginity and the story they tell themselves about the event and its meaning has implications for their view of themselves and sex itself afterwards (Carpenter, 2005). Some have said things about this milestone as simple as "It was fine." Others have commented that the experience was quite positive, enjoyable, or even empowering. Still others have felt that their first sexual experience was negative in some way. This may have been related to the physical experience of sex itself, the interpersonal connection that they found to be disappointing or hurtful, or the circumstances that were not what they hoped for. I have also worked with clients who reported that, though they felt positive or excited about their first experience of sex at the time, they looked back on it with regret over some aspect of it. In my clinical experience, this has most often been true of men and women who feel in hindsight that they became sexually active too young or with the wrong person. The nature of their first sex has often had ramifications for their subsequent choices about sex and their view of their sexuality in a way that has become a part of their overall sexual narrative.

Narratives of Sexual Functioning

An aspect of our sexual story that has implications over the course of the life span relates to what we tell ourselves about the physical and interpersonal meanings of sexual functioning (Carpenter & DeLamater, 2012). From the time our first sexual consciousness emerges, we internalize messages from family, peers, older youth we wish to emulate, the media, and the social world at large. These messages pertain to the sexual desirability of our body, as well as the normalcy of our sexual urges and the patterns of our arousal and functioning. Is our sexual appetite normal? Does our body respond the way it's supposed to? This all feeds into the dimension of our story that relates to our masculinity or femininity and whether or not we will be worthy and successful in the sexual realm.

When individuals struggle with some aspect of their sexual functioning, the concern this causes is often related not only to the way the dysfunction interferes with their sexual pleasure, but also to what it means about them and their sexuality in general as well as for their sexual relationships. This is an aspect of the sexual narrative that is often marked by stress. I have worked with clients, both men and women, whose difficulty achieving a state of arousal or orgasm, for example, has been a source of insecurity and feelings of inadequacy not only for them but for their partners as well. Note the ways in which we may make meaning of something like this. Perhaps there is "something wrong" with me as a man or woman. Maybe you are just not attracted to me and that is why you don't get aroused or climax. Perhaps I am sexually inadequate and that is why I can't satisfy you.

These same dynamics hold true for men with respect to their ability to achieve and maintain an erection. We invest the male erection with enormous significance not only for the specific purpose of sexual pleasure, but also as some measure of virility and the sexual desirability of both partners. Again, challenges in this area can lead to deep feelings of insecurity and inadequacy. The story of such a personal challenge fits into the wider social and cultural narrative that says that men should be able to get an erection on demand, and that they should be able to make that erection last as long as they wish before orgasm. We have built an entire sector of the pharmaceutical industry on our efforts to see to it. Yet, erectile difficulties are quite common, even in young men (Capogrosso et al., 2013; Mialon, Berchtold, Michaud, Gmel, & Suris, 2012). Male clients in their late teens and early 20s I have worked with have worried that there is something wrong with them as men when they have had difficulties getting an erection during a sexual encounter or have lost their erection even during sex. Through supportive exploration, we have usually discovered that the issue was related to some kind of anxiety, not even necessarily related to sex. At times, this concern has been about money, work, or some other stress that had them preoccupied and distracted during sex. At other times, there has been an interpersonal issue underlying the erectile problem, such as conflict or ambivalence with their partner. When necessary, I have encouraged clients to speak with their physician to rule out any organic cause for their sexual difficulty. From a narrative point of view what is most significant here is the meaning clients make of this kind of struggle either in themselves or their partner, and the story they elaborate about themselves and their sexuality because of it.

In midlife and in older adults, changes in the body and in patterns of sexual responsiveness are of course expectable, and can similarly be a source of some distress. The narrative of the sexual self evolves with the life course and right along with the body (Jen, 2017; Sandberg, 2013, 2016; Thomas & Thurston, 2016; Træen et al., 2017). Changes in patterns of desire, response, and stamina for example may at times be integrated into the story of men and women as a normal part of the aging process. Conversely, they may be a source of anxiety or feelings of loss of one's younger self, a self that was perhaps viewed as more virile or feminine.

It is common that the normal process of aging or the consequences of illness more typical of midlife and beyond bring changes to the experience of one's sexuality that can have a negative impact on functioning and the narrative of the self (Træen et al., 2017). Regardless of age, most people want to feel that they can continue to be sexually active as long as they are physically healthy enough to do so. Often, a conversation with one's physician is in order. I have worked with a number of older women, for example, who reported that the issue of normal vaginal dryness following menopause has made sex uncomfortable and that this has taken a negative toll on their sex life and their sense of self. I encouraged them to speak with their gynecologist who was able to help with this issue. By finding a solution that was effective and readily available, they allowed themselves to envision a different future to their sexual story.

A similar dynamic was seen in some older male clients who were grateful to have survived prostate cancer, but were nonetheless impacted by the sexual side effects of treatment. In some cases, a frank conversation with their urologist allowed them to consider options that made it possible to remain sexually active. Still other clients have found that, particularly in advanced age, the waning of their physical sexual capacity came to be less important compared to the ongoing experience of intimacy with their partner of which sex had always been an expression (Sandberg, 2013, 2016). Narrative is most interested in the meanings made of these moments of the life cycle and the way they impact the story of the subjects both individually and in relationship.

We have seen that the narrative of our sexuality begins to be shaped in the first moments of our life and continues to our final breath. Perhaps like no other aspect of our personhood, it touches every part of our self and our ability to enter into relationships with others, both genitally and non-genitally. The story of our sexuality grounds us in our body, mind, and spirit and connects us to the world around us. The recursive relationship between our own sexual narrative and the sociocultural context in which it is embedded helps shape our sense of sexuality in all its dimensions: gender expression, sexual orientation, sexual history, sexual functioning, and more. For us as clinicians, exploring the sexual narrative of our clients, and our own for that matter, is about allowing a profound dimension of the experience of the person before me to unfold and to be held with sensitivity and compassion. The nonexploitative, nonphysical kind of intimacy that the therapeutic relationship offers draws on our mutual capacity for connection, and offers us the opportunity to explore this deeply personal and meaningful dimension of the self in a way that may be healing and life giving.

Case Example

Brenda was 23 years old when I first met her. I recall what a striking impression she made when I went to greet her in the waiting room of the mental health clinic where I was working at the time. I called her by her first name, and as she rose from her chair, I could see that all eyes in the room were on her. She was a pretty young African-American woman. Her hair was long and thick. Though her appointment was at 10:00 a.m. and most people were dressed quite casually, Brenda looked like she was ready to go out for the evening. Her makeup was meticulous and centered on bright red lipstick. She wore a very short skirt and very high heels that made her quite tall. She had on a good deal of jewelry including a pair of very large hoop earrings. As she approached me, she smiled softly and said hello.

We settled into the first session and Brenda told me that she was coming to therapy "to deal with a lot of things." She described a mix of feelings including sadness, anxiety, and a sense of emptiness that she herself often found confusing. Though she tried to project an air of great poise and self-confidence, she usually felt just the opposite. "A lot of the time," she said, "I don't even think I really know who I am." In a way that contradicted her rather brash outward appearance, Brenda was soft-spoken, almost shy. She was also clearly very bright, thoughtful, and articulate.

Keep in mind that, throughout the course of therapy, the clinician is taking in and "listening to" all of their impressions about the client as well as how they are responding to the client internally. All of this is part of the story, and all of it is communicating something even if they're not sure what it means yet. In this instance, it was important to notice that what Brenda was telling me matched her demeanor, but was at odds with her outward self-presentation. So we take note of it, wonder what role this plays in the story as a whole, and keep paying attention.

As I got to know Brenda, a good deal of her narrative came to focus on her experience of her sexuality. She was raised by a single mother in a poor urban environment. It was just the two of them. Brenda reached puberty early and recalled only being 12 or 13 when she noticed men looking at her in a different way. Sometimes they were the teenage boys in the neighborhood; sometimes they were much older. They were men who hung out on the corner, lingered at the convenience store down the block, or just sat on the steps in front of their apartment buildings. From that early age, Brenda was aware not only of their stares as she walked past, but also of the comments made to each other and more and more to her directly. At times there were men who would do more than talk, daring to touch her, first holding her hand, resting a hand on her shoulder, and then touching her buttocks and even her breasts. At first she was terribly frightened. Later she felt as if she was becoming numb to it.

Brenda said that she knew her mother was aware of this, and had, in fact, seen it happen on more than one occasion. But she said nothing. On a few occasions, when their funds were running low just before her mother's pay day, she would ask Brenda to go down to the store and ask the owner for groceries on credit. "He likes you," she would say. "I see the way he looks at you." Brenda felt conflicted but did as her mother asked. When the store owner fondled her breast and rubbed himself against her, she felt as though she couldn't or at least shouldn't resist. Once her mother sent her to talk to the landlord to ask him to be patient since they were behind on their rent. He said he would wait. But he also exposed himself and asked Brenda to touch him—which she did. She was 14.

As time passed, Brenda grew somewhat accustomed to this sexual attention from men. She had not actually dated anyone, but had had sex on a number of occasions with several different men, most of them closer to her age, but not all. She had not prostituted herself, she assured me. There was never an exchange of money; but there was something less tangible. At times it was a favor or knowing there would be someone to give her a ride if she needed one. Other times, it was the sense that someone was looking out for her and had her back.

Another person who fit into this category for Brenda was a woman named Simone who lived in the neighborhood and whom she and her mother knew casually. By this time, Brenda was 16. Simone was in her early 30s. She was very friendly and would occasionally pay Brenda to run errands for her, or to babysit her two young children. Brenda would sometimes hang out in her apartment, especially if her mother wasn't home, but sometimes even if she was. One such evening, Brenda recalled being shocked. They were sitting at Simone's kitchen table talking when she leaned over and kissed Brenda deeply on the mouth. Stunned, Brenda said nothing. Nor did she move. Simone looked at her and kissed her again before returning to the conversation. Brenda said she felt very confused. She was used to sexual attention from men, but not from a woman, especially an older woman whom she thought of as a cross between a mother figure and a friend. She wondered if she should keep her distance after that, but also didn't want to lose the friendship. She liked Simone after all and had grown accustomed to the pocket money she earned from the errands and babysitting.

At some point not long after that, though Brenda couldn't remember exactly when, they were alone together in the Simone's apartment when she kissed Brenda again. This time, however, things progressed further when Simone asked Brenda to perform oral sex on her. Brenda has never done this, but after a good deal of hesitation agreed. Afterwards Simone performed oral sex on Brenda. This happened on several occasions, until after some time Brenda's conflicted feelings about it led her to distance herself from Simone and end the relationship.

She did eventually begin to date a young man she knew from school. She was attracted to him, but was aware that it was the first time she felt something more. She really liked him. Though it was clear he was attracted to her too, she felt that he was interested in something more from her. After they had been talking and spending time together for several weeks, she decided that she would have sex with him. She had had sex before, but in her mind this was different. In some sense, it felt to her as if it would be her first time. This would be special. Brenda grew somewhat tearful as she recalled the evening. It started off as kind of romantic, with food and talking. But when they began to have sex, the young man started to treat her roughly. He called her names she didn't want to repeat to me. When she asked him to slow down because she wasn't ready yet, he ignored her. She said that his roughness made the sex hurt since she wasn't even aroused. She began to cry quietly, she said. When he noticed, he laughed at her. He told her just to lie still so he could finish.

Brenda and I worked together to try to understand what all of this meant for her in the context of her reasons for coming to therapy to begin with—the sense of nervous sadness and emptiness that she said seemed to haunt her. What did this sexual story mean in the context of the overall narrative of her self and the feeling that she didn't even really know who she was? As I talked with Brenda about the history and nature of her experience of sexuality, I framed it as a narrative—a story. She said she had never thought about it that way, but was clearly reflecting on it as we sat together. I suggested that most stories have certain themes that run through them and invited Brenda to wonder about what the main themes of her sexual story were. What were the lessons of her story up to this point? These came to her fairly easily.

Brenda told me that she saw several themes in her sexual story; she had learned quite a few lessons along the way. Most people are users, she told me. Even if you think they are looking out for you, or care about you, they are really focused on what's good for them, on how you can please them. This was true, she felt, even of her mother who, Brenda said, didn't mind exploiting Brenda's sexuality for her own gain, especially as a young girl.

Exploring further, Brenda also identified that a dominant theme in her sexual narrative was that sex is power. From the first time she stood as a frightened girl in the back corner of the store down the street while the owner fondled her breasts in exchange for credit on groceries, she learned that her body and her sexuality could be used as a commodity. She felt that she continued to learn that lesson through the sexual experiences of her adolescence. Especially as she grew tougher on the inside, Brenda learned that she could sexualize situations in order to get her way, and that was true with both men and women. Things may not always turn explicitly sexual, but she had the power to seduce people, to charm them with her sexuality.

I asked Brenda if there was any theme in her story about the price of that power of seduction, namely the cost to herself. She knew that there was. Yes, sex was power; but it was also a burden. She could use her sexuality to get what she wanted or needed; she could use her body. Sometimes she even did it without thinking or even necessarily meaning to. She lived in a way that was hypersexualized, she thought. In a way that I meant to be gently supportive, I said, "Really? Do you feel that's true?" Without missing a beat, she replied, "Of course it's true! Look at me. Why else would I dress this way?" I was at once impressed and taken aback by Brenda's level of insight, and could see that she was moving to even deeper layers of her sexual narrative. "Tell me more," I said.

"Sex is really all I have. It's all people want me for." She paused for several moments, clearly in touch with something deep within her. "That's what I meant before when I said that sex is also a burden. It feels like something heavy that I have to wear on the outside. Like I have to carry it around with me all the time. I never know when I'm going to need it. But I don't really ever get to feel connected to anybody, like I really know them and they know me. Hell, I'm not sure if I even know myself at this point!"

By this time, Brenda and I had been working together for several months. Though I sensed that we had developed a very good therapeutic relationship, her comment about never feeling connected to anyone made me wonder how she felt about our relationship, different as it was from others in her life. I asked, "What is it like to come here and talk with *me* about all this? I'm guessing you've never said these things out loud before." She paused. "No, I haven't ... It's ok I guess." I waited.

Brenda went on. "I've never been in therapy before. This is different. It's good, I mean. But sometimes I do get nervous coming here."

"What makes you nervous?" I asked.

"I don't know. Wondering if you'll judge me maybe?" She sought to reassure or perhaps rescue me, "I haven't felt that way though." She continued, "Maybe it's also that I haven't really thought about these things. I came here to talk about how I feel, to try to figure out who I am. But that's scary! What if I can't figure it out? I feel like I kind of trust you, but what if all this takes me places that are too scary?"

"What do you think would happen?" I asked.

She looked at me and smiled. "Well, then I could just seduce you too if I wanted to."

In my sense of Brenda's transference to me, as well as my own countertransference, I was aware that there was at times something seductive about Brenda, not in her outward appearance, but in her way of interacting. It was somewhere between flirtatious and erotic without being explicitly either of those. Recall earlier when I commented that I was aware of the difference between Brenda's outward appearance and her demeanor and behavior. I suggested that it is important to be aware of such information and wonder about its meaning in the context of the overall narrative. This situation is similar. I knew that there was something seductive about Brenda. I could observe it and feel it. And I knew it meant something. The important thing therapeutically, I felt, was to neither collude with nor retreat from it. I needed to sit with it and contain it. It was important to stay "right there" in the appropriate therapeutic space with Brenda, neither returning seduction for seduction nor communicating that in any way I feared her sexuality and needed to avoid her.

This was never more true than when Brenda told me she felt she could just seduce me too if therapy became in some way too threatening for her. Think about it in the context of her sexual narrative. Brenda's story had been that sex is all she has and all anyone is interested in from her. An overarching theme had been that "sex is my power. It can help me find my way forward, get me out of a jam, and shield me when I am feeling vulnerable." That was her narrative. So, it was of the utmost importance that her experience of therapy, her experience of *me* as a therapist and as a man, contribute something different to the narrative and challenge the inevitability of the story line that had dominated her sense of self thus far.

I asked Brenda if that was what she wanted, to seduce me as a way of avoiding her feelings and the work she came to therapy to do. "Yes, at times," she said. "But no." That wasn't what she really wanted. Though the story of her sexuality and the role of sex had dominated Brenda's self-narrative for so long, we began purposefully to explore other parts of her self, specifically other interests, qualities, and even relationships that she realized had not been sexualized in the way she was used to. Part of this included reflecting on the therapeutic relationship and the way the story of what she was doing in therapy was helping her craft a different trajectory for the unfolding narrative of her self. The therapeutic space gave Brenda a place where she could name and explore the lessons she had learned and also experiment with what else was true for her and about her, as well as who she wanted to be. Her sexuality and even sex were and would always be a part of this to be sure. But therapy came to be about stretching the very narrow narrative frame that had so long constricted her view of her self and her world. Brenda was bright, thoughtful, and insightful. These qualities proved most valuable in the work she did. They allowed her to tune into the story she had told herself over time and begin to attend to things that were different. They allowed her to make choices that were freer, if at times frightening, about how she wanted to interact with others and even with herself.

Questions and Activities for Discussion and Further Reflection

1. In the beginning of this chapter I offer a perspective on sexuality as being about far more than the way we relate to and make use of our genitals. Rather, I suggest, sexuality lies at the heart of what it means to connect to oneself and others as a human person. How does this compare to the way you have viewed sexuality up to this point? Do you agree or disagree with this point of view? How so?
2. Consider reflecting on your own sexual story, the messages that you feel have been communicated to you about the nature of sexuality, and what these have meant for you personally.
3. As a class, discuss the theory of sexual scripting. You might read one or more of the articles cited in this chapter or others. Brainstorm together about the kinds of sexual scripts that you see operating in the social and cultural world around you, as well as the implications of these.
4. Reflect with your supervisor or as a class on what it would be like for you to explore in some depth the sexual narrative of your client. If you haven't encountered this situation yet in your work, use one of the clients described in the chapter. What do you imagine it would be like for you to sit with them and their sexual story? How comfortable or uncomfortable would you feel? What do you think makes this so?
5. Using the story of Brenda or Peter or any of the other vignettes in the chapter, role-play the interaction with one of you being the client and the other the social worker. You can use one pair to role-play in front of the class and allow the other students to listen and even support the clinician. Or you can break up into multiple teams role-playing simultaneously. Do not worry about sticking to the description of the case as I have given it to you. Sit with the story of the client. Listen for and explore the narrative. If it doesn't feel too premature, you can wonder together about how the narrative might develop in a further way that is healing.
6. In the study by Logie et al. (2015), a number of social work students identified feeling caught off guard by their client coming out to them. Not only were they unsure what to say or how to proceed, they were awakened to the bias that led many of them to presume that the client was heterosexual without even realizing it. Reflect on your own reaction to this study. What do you imagine it would have been like to be in their shoes with that client? How might you have responded to her? Can you bring to awareness any implicit biases you might hold? How might these affect your work? Tune into the way the social environment has impacted your own narrative about human sexuality in this regard.
7. Identify social policies that impact or are related to the area of human sexuality (e.g., gender, sexual orientation, health care). What are the social and cultural narratives that underlie those policies? Are there alternative or competing narratives that are part of the social and cultural dialogue?
8. Did any of the examples or stories in this chapter stand out to you in particular? If so, which ones? What in particular struck you about that narrative? Does it suggest anything to you about your own story or that of your clients?
9. Articulate for yourself your understanding of the most important factors for a social worker to keep when trying to attend to sexual narrative in our work with clients.

References

Anderson, K. M., & Hiersteiner, C. (2008). Recovering from childhood sexual abuse: Is a 'storybook ending' possible? *American Journal of Family Therapy, 36*(5), 413–424. https://doi.org/10.1080/01926180701804592

Barnett, M., & Scaramella, L. V. (2013). Mothers' parenting and child sex differences in behavior problems among African American preschoolers. *Journal of Family Psychology, 27*(5), 773–783. https://doi.org/10.1037/a0033792

Brown, G. L., Craig, A. B., & Halberstadt, A. G. (2015). Parent gender differences in emotion socialization behaviors vary by ethnicity and child gender. *Parenting: Science and Practice, 15*(3), 135–157. https://doi.org/10.1080/15295192.2015.1053312

Bruner, J. (1990). *Acts of meaning*. Cambridge, MA: Harvard University Press.

Bruner, J. (1991). The narrative construction of reality. *Critical Inquiry, 18*(1), 1–21.

Capogrosso, P., Colicchia, M., Ventimiglia, E., Castagna, G., Clementi, M. C., Suardi, N., ... Salonia, A. (2013). One patient out of four with newly diagnosed erectile dysfunction is a young man: Worrisome picture from everyday clinical practice. *Journal of Sexual Medicine, 10*, 1833–1841. https://doi.org/10.1111/jsm.12179

Carpenter, L. M. (2005). *Virginity lost: An intimate portrait of first sexual experiences*. New York: New York University Press.

Carpenter, L. M., & DeLamater, J. (Eds.). (2012). *Sex for life: From virginity to Viagra, how sexuality changes throughout our lives*. New York: New York University Press.

Cooke-Jackson, A., Orbe, M. P., Johnson, A. L., & Kauffman, L. (2015). Abstinence memorable message narratives: A new exploratory research study into young adult sexual narratives. *Health Communication, 30*(12), 1201–1212. https://doi.org/10.1080/10410236.2014.924045

Counselman, E. F. (2014). Containing and using powerful therapist reactions. In L. Motherwell & J. J. Shay (Eds.), *Complex dilemmas in group therapy: Pathways to resolution* (2nd ed., pp. 109–119). New York, NY: Routledge/Taylor & Francis Group.

Draucker, C. B., Martsolf, D. S., Roller, C., Knapik, G. P., Ross, R., & Stidham, A. W. (2011). Healing from childhood sexual abuse: A theoretical model. *Journal of Child Sexual Abuse: Research, Treatment, & Program Innovations for Victims, Survivors, & Offenders, 20*(4), 435–466. https://doi.org/10.1080/10538712.2011.588188

Fasula, A. M., Carry, M., & Miller, K. S. (2014). A multidimensional framework for the meanings of the sexual double standard and its application for the sexual health of young black women in the U.S. *Journal of Sex Research, 51*(2), 170–183. https://doi.org/10.1080/00224499.2012.716874

Foucault, M. (1978). *The history of sexuality: An introduction* (Vol. 1). New York: Vintage Books.

Foucault, M. (1979). *Discipline and punish*. New York: Vintage Books.

Gagnon, J. H., Rosen, R. C., & Leiblum, S. R. (1982). Cognitive and social aspects of sexual dysfunction: Sexual scripts in sex therapy. *Journal of Sex and Marital Therapy, 8*(1), 44–56.

Gagnon, J. H., & Simon, W. (1973). *Sexual conduct: The social sources of human sexuality*. Chicago: Aldine Books.

Gergen, K. J. (2015). *An invitation to social construction* (3rd ed.). Thousand Oaks, CA: Sage.

Grossman, F. K., Sorsoli, L., & Kia-Keating, M. (2006). A gale force wind: Meaning making by male survivors of childhood sexual abuse. *American Journal of Orthopsychiatry, 76*(4), 434–443.

Hammack, P. L., Thompson, E. M., & Pilecki, A. (2009). Configurations of identity among sexual minority youth: Context, desire, and narrative. *Journal of Youth and Adolescence, 38*, 867–883. https://doi.org/10.1007/s10964-008-9342-3

Hess, M., Ittel, A., & Sisler, A. (2014). Gender-specific macro- and micro-level processes in the transmission of gender role orientation in adolescence: The role of fathers. *European Journal of Developmental Psychology, 11*(2), 211–226. https://doi.org/10.1080/17405629.2013.879055

Jen, S. (2017). Older women and sexuality: Narratives of gender, age, and living environment. *Journal of Women & Aging, 29*(1), 87–97. https://doi.org/10.1080/08952841.2015.1065147

Kamya, H. (2012). The cultural universality of narrative techniques in the creation of meaning. In R. A. McMackin, E. Newman, J. M. Fogler, & T. M. Keane (Eds.), *Trauma therapy in context: The science and craft of evidence-based practice* (pp. 231–245). Washington, DC: American Psychological Association.

Krayer, A., Seddon, D., Robinson, C. A., & Gwilym, H. (2015). The influence of child sexual abuse on the self from adult narrative perspectives. *Journal of Child Sexual Abuse, 24*, 135–151.

Lamb, M. E., & Lewis, C. (2010). The development and significance of father-child relationships in two-parent families. In M. E. Lamb (Ed.), *The role of the father in child development* (pp. 94–153). Hoboken, NJ: John Wiley & Sons.

Logie, C. H., Bogo, M., & Katz, E. (2015). "I didn't feel equipped": Social work students' reflections on a simulated client "coming out". *Journal of Social Work Education, 51*(2), 315–328.

Masters, N. T., Casey, E., Wells, E. A., & Morrison, D. M. (2013). Sexual scripts among young heterosexually active men and women: Continuity and change. *Journal of Sex Research, 50*(5), 409–420.

Mialon, A., Berchtold, A., Michaud, P. A., Gmel, G., & Suris, J. C. (2012). Sexual dysfunctions among young men: Prevalence and associated factors. *Journal of Adolescent Health, 51*(1), 25–31. https://doi.org/10.1016/j.jadohealth.2012.01.008

Mitchell, K. R., Wellings, K., Nazareth, I., King, M., Mercer, C. H., & Johnson, A. M. (2011). Scripting sexual function: A qualitative investigation. *Sociology of Health & Illness, 33*(4), 540–553.

Montemurro, B. (2017). "The way that I look at things [is] different because it's me": Constructing and deconstructing narratives about racialized sexual selves. *Symbolic Interaction*. https://doi.org/10.1002/symb.300

Mossige, S., Jensen, T. K., Gulbrandsen, W., Reichelt, S., & Tjersland, O. A. (2005). Children's narratives of sexual abuse: What characterizes them and how do they contribute to meaning-making? *Narrative Inquiry, 15*(2), 377–404. https://doi.org/10.1075/ni.15.2.09mos

Saha, S., Chung, M. C., & Thorne, L. (2011). A narrative exploration of the sense of self of women recovering from childhood sexual abuse. *Counselling Psychology Quarterly, 24*(2), 101–113. https://doi.org/10.1080/09515070.2011.586414

Saketopoulou, A. (2011). Minding the gap: Intersections between gender, race, and class in work with gender variant children. *Psychoanalytic Dialogues, 21*, 192–209.

Sandberg, L. (2013). Just feeling a naked body close to you: Men, sexuality and intimacy in later life. *Sexualities, 16*(3–4), 261–282. https://doi.org/10.1177/1363460713481726

Sandberg, L. (2016). In lust we trust? Masculinity and sexual desire in later life. *Men and Masculinities, 19*(2), 192–208. https://doi.org/10.1177/1097184X15606948

Schauer, M., Neuner, F., & Elbert, T. (2011). *Narrative exposure therapy: A short-term treatment for traumatic stress disorders*. Cambridge, MA: Hogrefe.

Simon, W., & Gagnon, J. H. (2003). Sexual scripts: Origins, influences and changes. *Qualitative Sociology, 26*(4), 491–497.

Thomas, H. N., & Thurston, R. C. (2016). A biopsychosocial approach to women's sexual function and dysfunction at midlife: A narrative review. *Maturitas, 87*, 49–60. https://doi.org/10.1016/j.maturitas.2016.02.009

Træen, B., Hald, G. M., Graham, C. A., Enzlin, P., Janssen, E., Kvalem, I. L., … Štulhofer, A. (2017). Sexuality in older adults (65+)—An overview of the literature, part 1: Sexual function and its difficulties. *International Journal of Sexual Health, 29*(1), 1–10. https://doi.org/10.1080/19317611.2016.1224286

van der Pol, L. D., Groeneveld, M. G., van Berkel, S. R., Endendijk, J. J., Hallers-Haalboom, E. T., Bakermans-Kranenburg, M. J., & Mesman, J. (2015). Fathers' and mothers' emotion talk with their girls and boys from toddlerhood to preschool age. *Emotion, 15*(6), 854–864. https://doi.org/10.1037/emo0000085

White, M., & Denborough, D. (2011). *Narrative practice: Continuing the conversations*. New York, NY: W W Norton & Company.

Zaman, W., & Fivush, R. (2013). Gender differences in elaborative parent–child emotion and play narratives. *Sex Roles, 68*(9–10), 591–604. https://doi.org/10.1007/s11199-013-0270-7

Chapter 6
Leaving Home, Finding Home: Narrative Practice with Immigrant Populations

Guiding Questions

What does narrative theory have to offer as a way of understanding the immigration experience?
How does narrative theory inform our practice with individuals, families, and communities who have lived an immigration experience?
What are the phases of the immigration experience and what do each of these contribute to the meaning it holds for those who live it?
What kinds of losses are immigrants likely to experience and how do these contribute to the development of the immigration story?
What are the social, cultural, and political voices that contribute to the shaping of our collective narratives of immigration? How do these voices impact the lived experience of immigrants and the communities in which they live?

There is perhaps no topic that is more timely in both American and international discourse, nor one that is capable of provoking such heated divisions between us as immigration. As I write this, the news is peppered on a daily basis with accounts of people on the move. These stories are communicated in words and images, and seem to come from every perspective imaginable. We listen to the voices of politicians, advocates, human rights and relief workers, and sometimes of immigrants themselves. Narratives are woven about the impetus for these migrations, and the intentions of those involved. Whether the movements of immigrants around the world are greeted with compassion, suspicion, or outright fury is largely a function of the tales that are told about their motivations, honest or nefarious, and the sense we have of our own and others' responsibility toward these individuals, families, and even ethnic groups.

The story of immigration is not a singular one. In some ways it is true to say that there are as many immigration narratives as there are immigrants. Yet journalism and social science scholarship in this area do allow us to identify and reflect on common trends in these stories, and there is much we know about the reasons people migrate, the experiences they have along the way, and the impact of the reception they receive when they arrive and settle into a new land. We are also fortunate to be able to look at the narrative structure and function of the stories we tell each other and ourselves about immigrants and immigration. The aim of this chapter is to examine, through the lens of narrative, the nature of the immigration experience from the point of view of both immigrants themselves and the social, cultural, and political environments that surround them.

Let's begin by setting the stage with some current data about the state of immigration in the United States and around the world. According to the Pew Research Center, in 2015 the foreign-born population of the United States was 43.2 million (Lopez & Bialik, 2017). This is an all-time high and four times the US immigrant population of 50 years earlier in 1965. The Pew Center offers further details. Seventy-six percent of these immigrants are authorized to live in the United States while the remaining 24% are not. Forty-four percent of those individuals born outside the United States have since become US citizens. In 1990, unauthorized immigrants numbered 3.5 million. In 2015, there were 11 million, down by just over a million from 2007. The drop between 2007 and 2015 largely occurred among Mexican immigrants, while the United States saw an influx of people arriving from Central America, Asia, and sub-Saharan Africa. The United States continues to see a rise of approximately one million immigrants each year, most notably from Asia. Since 1980, and included in the overall foreign-born population, the United States has admitted approximately three million refugees, 84,995 of whom entered in 2016 (Lopez & Bialik, 2017).

The United Nations High Commission on Refugees (UNHCR) has recently offered some powerful statistics regarding the state of refugees around the world. As of June 2017, the UNHCR reports that 65.6 million individuals have been displaced from their home, 20 displaced forcibly every minute, while 22.5 million are identified as refugees (United Nations High Commission on Refugees, 2017). Additionally, the UNHCR reports that ten million people are stateless and live without the basic human rights typically afforded by citizenship. In other words, they are not recognized as the legal citizens of any country and thus are not guaranteed protection by anyone (United Nations High Commission on Refugees, 2017).

Take a moment now, and ask yourself what all these statistics say to you. What is the message you hear in them? Don't take this interpretation for granted, and understand that there are a variety of ways that different individuals, group, and governments make sense of them. Do these numbers tell a tale of a border problem that is out of control? Do they speak of humanitarian crisis or a worldwide struggle for a better life? Do they suggest an opportunity for those who intend us harm to exploit holes in the system and draw ever closer? Do they tell of a persistent pattern of global violence perpetrated by those who either seek to exploit human life for their own gain or at the very least are blind to the suffering they cause? In that story, are we as a country weak, compassionate, heartless, calculating, understandably self-protective? Does the story call us to defend our border? Does it compel us to bring relief and offer support? Perhaps your interpretation is some combination of these and even other story lines.

If narrative does nothing else, it tunes us into the complexity of the world around us, and urges us to be clear and critical in evaluating the sources and meanings of the messages we hear every day as well as the sense we make of them. With respect to immigration, these messages touch us and shape us individually and collectively (Bruner, 1986, 1990, 1991). As in other areas of our life, they bridge the inner and outer worlds as we seek to make sense of what is happening around us and ascribe meaning to our lived experience.

The Narrative of the Journey: Stories of Flight and Promise

All narratives of immigration tell the story of a journey. Immigration is not about the moment or means of crossing a border from one country to another (Sowards & Pineda, 2013). It is not about any single moment or motivation. Of necessity, like all narratives, these stories unfold over time and are made up of phases and transitions, each of which has something to say about the one that precedes it and the one that follows. Foster (2001) described a framework that is useful in conceptualizing the phases of the immigration journey. Though she is writing specifically about the nature of immigration trauma, the overall understanding of the stages of the journey is useful for our beginning discussion here.

According to Foster (2001), the narrative of immigration begins in the country of origin. There are a host of factors that contribute to the nature and meaning of this part of the story. What were the conditions in the home country or the personal circumstances of the individual that led to the decision to emigrate? This is an essential consideration that contributes the "why" to the immigration narrative. For some, this may involve circumstances of violence and oppression that they felt necessitated their departure. This may be related to the political climate in their country (Fortuna, Porche, & Alegria, 2008) or may relate to something more personal such as the culture's rejection of someone of their religion (Grim & Finke, 2011) or sexual orientation (Alessi, 2016; Portman & Weyl, 2013). For others, the impetus to leave may be related to economic circumstances or the promise of a better life elsewhere.

Additionally, the narrative of a person's immigration is influenced by factors such as the haste with which they left, how much they were able to plan and prepare, and whether or not they were able to say goodbye. Consider that for some immigrants their story includes memories of a bon voyage party and the well wishes of family and friends. For others, it involves fleeing with a word to no one under cover of darkness.

The second phase of the immigration story pertains to the journey to the new land and how this was undertaken. Consistent with what I just noted about the departure, these narratives are shaped by whether they began in an international airport as a planned journey, or by other means that may be far more treacherous.

Consider this, for example. In his book, Strength in What Remains, Kidder (2010) tells the true story of Deogratias (Deo), a medical student from Burundi, forced to flee on foot through the jungle when a civil war and genocide erupted between the Hutus and Tutsis. After a harrowing journey during which his life was threatened at every turn, Deo finally reached the hoped for safety of Rwanda, only to find that the genocide spread quickly and even more famously through that country as well. After months of struggling to survive, Deo boarded an airplane bound for New York and the hope of a better life that awaited him, but the ghosts of that journey haunted him for some time to come.

Here is a different example. Many years ago, I lived and worked in an inner-city community where I was fortunate to be befriended by an extended family of immigrants from Mexico. The family consisted of several sisters, their husbands, and their children. Only one of the sisters and her husband were authorized to live in the United States. The others lived in fear of discovery and deportation, but they said that the risk was worth it because the conditions of poverty in their village in Mexico were so severe that a life there with their children was unimaginable. Each of the adults held several jobs, mostly in restaurants and factories. They worked in alternating shifts so that those who were off could take care of all the children. They were a close-knit, hard-working, loving family. They had a quiet, humble demeanor and largely kept to themselves except for a circle of friends they had mostly met at their church.

One day when I had been invited to dinner, I sat talking with Milagros, one of the sisters. I was close enough to the family that they had talked with me about their concerns regarding deportation and the impossibility of returning home. Milagros said, "Have I ever told you the story of how I came here?" She hadn't, I replied. "We had made arrangements for the coyote [a contractor who will transport people illegally across the border for an often high and sometimes uncertain price] to bring me and the eldest of the children across the border." Milagros recounted how she was instructed to arrive at a warehouse at a certain location before dawn. The spot was isolated and unlikely to attract unwanted attention. It was about 30 miles from the US/Mexican border. She was there early, as were a number of other people whom she could see moving about in the darkness. No one spoke. No one stood together. Yet they all knew the common motivation that brought them there.

Before long, the coyote arrived with another man in a large box truck. As the truck entered the warehouse, everyone followed in silence. The coyote and his partner proceeded to open the box truck and remove what turned out to be its false floor. This revealed a shallow empty compartment that covered the area of the truck's bottom. The two men instructed those present that they would lie in the bottom, and would be covered by the false floor. The truck would be loaded with boxes in case they were stopped along the way or at the border for inspection. Once they crossed the border, they would stop at an isolated location where they would be freed from the truck and could be on their way.

As Milagros told me the story I could see her struggling to catch her breath, much as she told me she did on that morning. Milagros and her daughter approached the truck when they were told it was their turn. In order to accommodate as many people as possible, everyone was required to lie on their side. This resulted in Milagros lying almost nose-to-nose with a strange man facing her. She could feel his breath on her cheek. Her young daughter lay pressed between them. When the false floor was put in place, Milagros said that she could feel her shoulders being pressed together—an effect that only worsened as boxes were loaded onto the truck.

The temperature rose quickly and soon came to feel almost unbearable. Wrapped in the darkness of the compartment, with strangers packed in around her, the truck began to move, each bump as frightening as it was jolting. The rumble of the engine and the grind of the transmission, now only inches beneath her, were deafening. Milagros told of feeling near panic, wondering if she would ever make it out of that truck, if she would really be free to move on to her future, uncertain as it was. She recalled holding her breath when the slow roll of the truck and frequent braking told her that they were at the border. Soon the engine was shut off and she heard the sound of men's voices in the distance as the drivers presented their papers and spoke to the border and customs agent. Like her fellow passengers, she was almost holding her breath in an effort to make no noise. A muffled cough rose here, the whimper of a small child there.

After a prolonged wait that she felt certainly meant they were caught, the engine started, the gears of the transmission ground into place, and the truck began to roll again. Some time later, she couldn't tell how long, the truck stopped. Milagros said that when the last box was removed and the floor was finally lifted, she cried with relief. Nonetheless, she knew her journey wasn't done. It was only after a walk of several hours through the desert and several days worth of bus rides that she and her daughter were at last reunited with her sister in New York, and she was able to wonder what kind of new life lay ahead.

This leads us to the third phase of the immigration journey and narrative. Though not experienced by all who migrate to another country, this stage involves a temporary detainment in some settlement or facility designed for the processing of newly arrived immigrants. In past generations, Ellis Island served such a purpose for the millions of new arrivals coming to the United States through New York. Depending on one's health (arrivals were examined and tested for disease) and the circumstances of one's arrival, one might be released from Ellis Island quite quickly or be detained for some time. A small number were even turned away.

In places around the world, even large groups of immigrants are housed in camps and detention centers for extended periods of time (Foster, 2001). This may be related to delays in considering requests for admission to the host country, the difficulty of assimilating large number of arrivals (especially in countries that are economically struggling), or both. For those who are seeking asylum status in the United States, such detention centers amount to incarceration for undetermined periods of time and without due process while one's application is considered.

A word of clarification is in order here regarding the difference between a refugee and an asylee (i.e., someone seeking asylum), at least in the context of US law (U.S. Citizenship and Immigration Services, 2015). Though policy and procedure in this area are highly complex, consider this distinction. Both refugees and asylees are people who have fled their country of origin due to persecution or fear of persecution over things such as their religion, ethnic identity, membership in a particular social group, and political affiliation. Refugees are recognized as such and arrive in their new country with that status. By contrast, those seeking asylum arrive without refugee status. They may then apply for asylum status and may be detained while their application is reviewed. What are the implications of this distinction? Because of their recognized status, refugees are permitted to work upon their arrival in the United States and are also entitled to receive public benefits. In addition to the possibility of prolonged detention, asylees are usually not permitted to work and are not eligible for public benefits.

Whether in refugee camps or detention centers, these individuals, families, and sometimes whole communities are fleeing violence, abuse, or a humanitarian crisis of some kind and during their transition often endure overcrowding, conflict, fear, and unsanitary conditions. For these men, women, and children, it is important to acknowledge that migration means journeying *from* more than *to* (Hollander, 2006). The primary goal is getting distance from the harmful situation in which they found themselves. For this reason, the otherwise awful circumstances of these camps or centers are considered preferable to a return to those from which they came.

The fourth phase of the immigration experience involves the ultimate resettlement in the host country and the nature of the specific environment in which that takes place. This dimension of the story is, to one extent or another, a part of the narrative of all immigrants regardless of how they came to be in their new environment. Though in some sense it may seem that the journey is over, there is still more that awaits the newly arrived. Imagine yourself having just settled in a place that you hope will offer you the promise of safety, or a better life for yourself and your family. Imagine that you have fled the violence of war or persecution. Imagine that you have made a planned move to a new country for the purposes of work, or the pursuit of opportunity. Consider the almost innumerable variables that will condition the nature of your experience and impact the way you process it: language, food, physical environment, safety, climate, living conditions, availability and suitability of work, financial sustainability, comprehension of the nuances of what is happening in the culture around you, and emotional tone of the reception you are given by the host community. The taken-for-grantedness of so much of your environment is overturned such that, even if you are profoundly grateful to be here, you are likely overwhelmed, disoriented, and struggling to get your bearings.

Many years ago, American friends of mine, a husband and wife, moved to the West Indies in the Caribbean to work in community development with a nongovernmental organization. In many ways their new life seemed enviable, like a permanent vacation. The weather was beautiful. They woke every morning to views of the sea. They could swim in any number of nearby streams and rivers, not to mention the Caribbean itself any time they wished, and take evening walks on the beach. It sounded fantastic, and in some ways it was. I was fortunate enough to go for a visit, and we talked about what it was like to move from the United States to this tropical island. All the wonderful things were in fact wonderful. At the same time, they talked about what it was like to get "island fever", to feel almost suffocated by the awareness that you were on an island—completely surrounded by water. Though that island was 30 miles long and there was obviously enough space, they began to feel claustrophobic, knowing that the only way out was by plane or boat.

Though they respected the community and hoped to make a positive contribution through their presence and work, they talked about not feeling welcomed by some of the locals who had a less than positive view of Americans. In fact, there was at times some open hostility. They were called names based on their race, and told to go back where they came from. As white Americans, the irony did not escape them that they were getting a taste of what so many racial and ethnic minorities and immigrants had experienced in the United States.

Over time they found themselves sorely missing things that were familiar and meaningful to them even without their realizing it. These things had been taken for granted until they were no longer there. For example, they told me about their first experience of a Caribbean Christmas. Christmas happened to be one of their favorite holidays and though they planned on returning to the United States for a visit later that winter they chose to remain on the island for the holiday itself. Just like in the United States, there was a lot of buildup to Christmas on the island with a local festival, parties, shopping, and the like. After talking with some of the members of the local community with whom they had become friends, they had planned the events of the day together. For the first time in their lives, they didn't have a Christmas tree. There were no pine trees on the island, and no pop-up tree lots where they could go purchase their tree like they had done together for so many years. They attended a Church service together in the morning, but were surprised to realize that they knew none of the songs. Instead of the "traditional" Christmas songs with which they were familiar, the songs they heard had a Calypso style that was really beautiful, though they had never heard the tunes or the words before. No one used music books because they knew the words by heart. So my friends listened and followed along.

After Church they went home where they changed into shorts and flip-flops. They gathered their bathing suits and towels and headed to the beach where they were meeting friends. The weather was really beautiful and the water was perfect. Later they went back to their friends' home and joined their family celebration. They had prepared goat especially for Christmas dinner. It was traditional for the family, and my friends did happen to like goat. For dessert there was a traditional Christmas rum cake, with plenty of rum of course.

Looking back on the day as they talked with me about it, they said it was a beautiful Christmas celebration, but one that also highlighted for them how alone and out of place they felt in many ways. They were grateful to have made some wonderful friends who received them with real warmth and included them like family in the celebration. And there was an excitement in the newness and difference of it all. But they were also keenly aware of all that they were missing. Christmas is supposed to be cold, if not snowy. Christmas features a big tree in the living room, covered with ornaments. Christmas is wool sweaters, not bathing suits. It is deciding whether to have turkey or ham for dinner, not goat no matter how delicious it is. Christmas is the traditional carols they had learned as children and sang every year.

It is very possible that as you read this you are saying something like "Wait a second. That isn't my idea of Christmas. I live in Florida or Hawaii and I've gone to the beach plenty of times on Christmas. And we never eat turkey or ham. We have lamb." And maybe you don't celebrate Christmas at all. A good friend of mine who is Jewish has a very regular Christmas tradition. She and her family go to the movies and then go out for Chinese food. All of this is, of course, the point. Whatever the reason for our being in a different country or a different culture, so much of what we take for granted, even the way we celebrate our favorite holiday, may be called into question. With that in mind, let us consider in some greater depth the nature of loss and its impact on the immigration narrative.

Loss and the Potential for Growth in the Immigration Narrative

We have seen that each stage of the journey of immigration can bring with it its own stressors, beginning with the separation from one's homeland to the effort to adapt to a new environment (Hollander, 2006). There is ample evidence in the scholarly literature regarding the way that this process of transition may be marked by numerous losses (Ainslie, Tummala-Narra, Harlem, Barbanel, & Ruth, 2013; Akhtar, 1995; Tummala-Narra, 2014). Even beyond the loss of material possessions that one could not bring on the journey, these kinds of losses may seem less visible and for that reason be less immediately recognized. For us as clinicians, however, it is deeply important that we be aware of the many ways immigrant clients and communities may be challenged. These changes, whether stark or subtle, can impact the narrative of immigrants in profound ways. Like all losses, these involve some degree of mourning as well as a renegotiation of one's sense of self and the world.

Perhaps one of the most fundamental losses experienced by many immigrants is language. Be aware of the fact that narrative is cast in language. We are always formulating our personal narrative in the language that is most intimately available to us, our so-called mother tongue (Mirsky, 1991). This is the language in which we speak to ourselves in the privacy of our minds, the language of our dreams.

Language is about more than the words we use to name things. This can be confusing enough on its own—having to search for the words for even the simplest items we need or the most straightforward questions or ideas we wish to express, or knowing that the word may not even be there to be found. Even more deeply, however, language has affective meaning. It is the tool we use to give shape to our most basic sense of self and the world—like a sculptor who uses clay or marble or metal to give form to his or her vision.

In the early 1990s I had the opportunity to spend a few months in the Dominican Republic where my main goal was to learn Spanish. I had studied Spanish before and when I arrived I could, as they say, "defend myself." That is, I could get along with the basics and maybe a bit more, but just a bit. I was participating in an immersion program where I had four hours of private tutoring every day, and changed teachers every two weeks. Perhaps the best part of the program, however, was that I lived with a family in the neighborhood. They were a married couple, Claudio and Juana, with two small children. One of the husband's nieces had also come from the *campo* (the country) to live with them and help with housework and childcare. They were a lovely family and took great care of me. And I enjoyed living with them. As my Spanish improved, I was able to spend time with Claudio and Juana in the evening talking about everything from Dominican history and culture to politics and their perceptions of life in the United States. Claudio started to tell me jokes in Spanish, speaking slowly, helping me to understand the words and, what is so often key to a good joke, the play on words. At times I just couldn't get it, and with a laugh he would break it down and explain it to me. But more and more I understood and would laugh in all the right places.

Claudio and Juana were sophisticated, highly educated people. Claudio was a child psychologist; Juana was a librarian in a school. After I had been with them for some time, they proposed that just as they were helping me with my Spanish perhaps I could help them a bit with their English. I agreed enthusiastically. I was happy to help them. It turned out that this was probably more of a learning experience for me than it was for them. I remember how struck I was, as they began to speak English with me, at the dramatic difference in their speech. These two articulate, insightful people sat with me and struggled simply to pronounce the words of even the most basic questions or statements about themselves. I remembered growing up in my multiethnic neighborhood in Brooklyn, and all the disparaging things I ever heard grown-ups say about ignorant immigrants who couldn't speak English. It never occurred to these adults that they could not speak a word of Spanish or Creole or Chinese or any language other than English for that matter. Consider every immigrant who has ever been told that if they want to live here they should speak English or go home. Think of every time you have heard an immigrant struggling to speak English and the story you have told yourself of what that meant about them.

The effort to express oneself in a foreign language can cut to the core of the story one tells about one's self, and one's competence and abilities. The shift in that narrative can come from not only the change of language itself, but also the consequences this can have in one's life. I've met an Arabic-speaking man from the Middle East who was a physicist working as a school janitor because he could only speak the most basic English, a Latin American physician and medical school professor who took a job in a factory because it would not have been possible for her to take the licensing exams in a foreign language, and an attorney who left behind her career and did childcare out of her apartment. Each of them had their own reasons why coming to the United States was worth it, in spite of this loss. But this did not mean the loss was any less real.

There are a few different dimensions of this experience that I think are worth examining from a narrative point of view. Each of these individuals had to cope with a radical challenge to their self-narrative as they saw their social position change from middle/upper class professional to a service worker barely earning enough to get by (Hollander, 2006). Furthermore, they dealt with the humbling and sometimes humiliating experience of seeing their status reduced in the eyes of the society around them. This ranged from sensing blatant hostility, to feeling invisible to the eyes of those who presumed themselves to be better than a poor immigrant, to the well meaning but unknowing response of even those who wished them well. Additionally, I suggest that it is essential for us as social workers to understand whatever implicit biases we bring to these encounters. These include the story we tell ourselves about the immigrants and immigrant communities we encounter, as well as the varied narratives about immigrants to which we are all exposed in the culture at large.

As an extension of this, we must be mindful in the design and delivery of clinical services of the importance of offering as much as possible the opportunity for people to receive services in their own language, and from someone who understands not only vocabulary but also culture. It is semantically and emotionally limiting if not impossible to express the deepest and most sensitive aspects of one's narrative in a language that is not one's own, that cannot be felt on a visceral level, and that does not capture the affective resonance of one's experience.

Beyond the fundamental kind of loss that may be related to issues of language, immigrants trying to adapt to a new environment are also challenged to deal with differences in the social story that conveys cultural norms and values. Once again, consider the taken-for-granted nature of so many of these assumptions that are implicit in our narratives and that only come to the fore when they are challenged by difference. Here I am referring to issues such as what is considered proper behavior in any number of social situations. What do our nonverbal behaviors mean, and how are we to interpret them? What is the expected pace of life in the place you live? Do you ever find someone moving too slowly, or too quickly for your liking? What do you imagine about those people? How does this relate to your sense of time and the importance of time? Even within the United States, for example, there is wide variation regionally in how these aspects of life are lived, and we tell ourselves stories about what people from this or that part of the country are like and what life there is all about. But now consider the perspective of a Syrian refugee or an adolescent from Calcutta who arrives in a small Midwestern town, or downtown Los Angeles.

We may also think of nonverbal forms of communication and the narrative they suggest. Pay attention, for example, to the way we interpret facial expressions and body language. How do we use them to express, consciously or unconsciously, messages such as openness or defensiveness, fear or aversion versus interest and an invitation to draw closer? How do we use physical space, particularly the space between people? This is the study of what is known as *proxemics* (Hall, 1963) and it often tells a very clear story about people and their expectations. There are cultures for example where it is customary to stand quite close together while speaking. Greater distance might be seen as rude or off-putting. Conversely, in a culture that places greater value on personal space, standing close might feel aggressive or otherwise intrusive. Think about the way that this kind of experience might shape the story we tell about the other and the meaning of their behavior. The same observation may be made about the volume of one's speech, and the meaning of maintaining or avoiding direct eye contact (Matsumoto, 2006). For many immigrants who have come from more homogenous societies, they may find themselves "raced" for the first time, and have to deal with unfamiliar stereotypes and biases projected onto them based on the others' perception of their race. Tummala-Narra (2014), for example, writes of a client from Jamaica who came to the United States and was referred to for the first time as "African-American." Not having any identification with Africa at all, and never having thought of herself this way in the context of her Jamaican culture, the client found this surprising.

Within the structure of a family, challenges to the expected narrative may surface in a number of ways. For immigrant families, the potential for conflict between their own cultural norms and expectations and those of the host culture, may be significant. Imagine a multigenerational family, including grandparents, parents, and children, that immigrates to another country. While traditional wisdom has been that children will acculturate more quickly than their parents, this may not always be so (Nieri et al., 2016). Each family should be assessed to understand its own story and process. Nonetheless, differences in the pace of acculturation and the challenge this represents to the traditional family narrative can be a source of distress for everyone involved (Arbona et al., 2010). I have known families, for example, in which parents and grandparents struggled with competing narratives. They simultaneously told the story of how their children would adjust, feel at home, and build a future for themselves in their new country, as well as the story of how they would remain faithful to their native culture and traditions. They then felt upset when they saw their children or grandchildren becoming "too Americanized," turning their back on their family duties in a way that sometimes even felt disrespectful.

For their part, these children or teens felt caught in the middle, making their way in their new environment, learning a new way of understanding the world, while also having to comply with traditions from which they felt increasingly far removed. This clash of narratives can lead to resentments and family conflict and needs to be understood for what it is and worked through. I have known quite a number of young women from immigrant families who were told, often explicitly, that they must work hard in university and do well, but that they were also expected to home by 3 o'clock every afternoon to take care of the younger children, help clean around the house, and prepare the evening meal. These dueling responsibilities emerged from well-intentioned but conflicting stories about the role of a responsible and respectful young woman in her family, and put these young ladies in an inevitable bind.

The issue of gender-based narratives can present even further difficulties for immigrant families. It is not uncommon for immigrants to come to a new country only to find that the gender roles that have been an expected part of their cultural narrative get turned on their heads. This may be related both to general differences between the culture of origin and the host culture, and to the exigencies of the particular situation in which the family members find themselves. Imagine a family coming to a large North American city from a country where the roles of men and women are sharply divided. Women take care of the home and children. Men go out into the world, work, and provide for the family. It is important to note that this belief system may be a by-product not only of their culture but also of their social class, which also helps shape their narrative.

In the North American context, they may struggle with the commonality with which both men and women work outside the home (particularly in the most expensive parts of the country where two incomes are often indispensable), and may find themselves needing to follow suit in order to live, thus challenging an aspect of the gender-based narrative on which they have relied. They may also be confronted with an outright reversal of roles if one or more of the females are able to find work and the men are not. This may require the men to care for the home and children or to leave all the responsibility to the women, either scenario being a great source of potential conflict. These same concerns, along with stories that cast men in the role of chief provider, exist in traditional North American gender narratives as well, of course. For newly immigrated families, however, they add yet another component to the upheaval into which they have been thrust and to which they have to adjust (Dion & Dion, 2001; Lindsey, 2015).

The kinds of phenomena we are examining are so numerous and varied that it might be difficult even to name them all. What's more, these attitudes often intersect with other forces of oppression in our society that keep members of immigrant groups marginalized (Tummala-Narra, 2014; Viruell-Fuentes, Miranda, & Abdulrahim, 2012). My hope is that you are tuning into the way in which all of these factors contribute to shaping the narrative we tell about ourselves and the other. This is as true of the perspective of the immigrant as it is the social environment into which they are received. Let's take a deeper look at the nature of identity and the narrative of the immigrant.

Renegotiating Identity: The Narrative of the Immigrant Self

The upheaval involved in the process of immigration requires a renegotiation to a greater or lesser extent of the immigrant's narrative of the self. Akhtar (1995) delineates a range of factors that contribute to the outcome of this renegotiation. They include whether the move to a new country is considered temporary or permanent, whether one had a choice in leaving one's country or was compelled to do so, whether the possibility of visiting the homeland exists, one's age at the time of migration, the positive or negative meaning of the reasons one has chosen to immigrate, one's psychological capacity to tolerate separateness at the time of immigration, the emotional tone of the host country's reception, the extent to which the cultures of the home and host countries differ, and the extent to which one can continue in one's role or profession upon arrival in the new country.

All of these factors, and perhaps even more, contribute to the degree of culture shock experienced by the immigrant as he or she engages in a process of acculturation, one which is by nature stressful. Arbona et al. (2010) suggest that acculturative stress "refers to the emotional reaction triggered by the individual's appraisal of specific events and circumstances in their lives" (p. 364). In other words, acculturative stress is our emotional response to the narrative we construct about the meaning of our experience. This stress is related to the immigrants' connection with both the home country and the host country, and may be aggravated by factors such as undocumented status (Nieri et al., 2016). Additionally, the impact of this stress may be felt both outside the family and within the family (Arbona et al., 2010), manifesting itself not only in family conflict, but also in reduced closeness and possibly ineffective parenting (Nieri et al., 2016).

As you can see, there is a wide range of factors and conditions that contribute to the unique construction of the immigrant's sense of their identity and to the renegotiation of that identity sparked by the immigration journey. In keeping with Arbona's (2010) view of acculturative stress, the way in which identity is renegotiated and the story is told about the nature of the immigration experience is conditioned on the very subjective appraisal of the immigrant himself or herself. You may recall that in Chap. 1, I discussed Spence's (1982) view of the distinction between narrative truth and historical truth. What is at play here is not an "objective" historical analysis by a dispassionate observer of events as they unfolded. Rather, it is the highly personalized story of a life experience and the meaning it holds for the crafter and teller of that story.

Benish-Weisman's (2009) study of 22 émigrés from the former Soviet Union to Israel revealed a great deal about the relationship between the immigrants' appraisal of their experience and the way they crafted that narrative. Her analysis of participant narratives found that those who view their immigrant experience as successful told stories that were coherent and well structured. This type of story form suggests a high degree of well-being and adjustment to one's new country, she suggests. Conversely, those who looked negatively on their immigration and saw it as unsuccessful produced narratives that were fragmented and lacked coherence. These were more suggestive of experiences of regression and defeat.

Benish-Weisman draws on Gergen and Gergen's (1988) typology of genres of such stories, including romance, comedy, and tragedy, that are reflective of the movement of the story from high points to low points or vice versa. However, she also describes two other patterns not accounted for in Gergen and Gergen's work but found in her subjects' narratives—namely, fracture and victimization. Fracture, she states, is characteristic of a story marked by deterioration and fragmentation. Victimization is seen in stories that are circular and repetitive, leading to a negative end and manifesting the author's perceived lack of control. Benish-Weisman (2009) also suggests that the relationship between episodes in the narrative may be characterized by patterns of redemption or contamination. The former is associated with the movement of the story from bad times to good, from hardship to success. Conversely, the contamination pattern reflects a movement from good (or at least better) to worse. It is clear that a redemption pattern is more likely to be found in a success story and is more suggestive of the author's well-being and positive adjustment.

With respect to stories of fracture, victimization, and contamination, Volkan (2007) offers a perspective on the way such unresolved narratives of loss can lead to their tellers becoming what he refers to as perennial mourners. Ethnic and other groups may attach themselves to a narrative of what was lost to them or what was taken from them individually and collectively. Volkan suggests that this may evolve into an ideology of entitlement wherein the members of the group maintain a focus on the restoration of all that they believe is rightfully theirs. This involves more than nostalgia or even longing. Rather, it is an investment that can result in ongoing mourning on the part of the individual and the group.

On a societal level, this may be manifested in the construction of memorials and monuments as well as the establishment of particular days of observance. What's more, the legacy of this loss may be passed on to subsequent generations who will become the bearers of this narrative in very particular ways. It is clear that this memory and mourning can serve an important social function. Who could imagine allowing the meaning and lessons of the Holocaust to fade from our collective consciousness? Following 9/11 one of the most common slogans to appear on memorials of all kinds was "Never Forgotten." However, for groups such as the children of Holocaust survivors and other genocides, it is also important to be attentive to the ways in which these narratives are carried at times as burdens on personal and social levels, as well as the impact not only of remembering but also of actively mourning across generations (Azarian-Ceccato, 2010).

So what does all this mean for us? The way we think of ourselves (successful or unsuccessful, capable or inept, etc.) bears a direct connection to the stories we tell ourselves and others *about* ourselves and the nature of our experience. As we all do in different arenas, immigrants elaborate a narrative of their journey in all its complexity that gives form and structure to the meaning they make of that experience.

From a developmental point of view, the renegotiation of identity that takes place through the immigration journey has been compared to the separation individuation processes that are part of childhood and adolescence. Mahler (1963), and Mahler, Pine, and Bergman (1975) described the separation individuation process whereby the toddler begins to explore the world and establish independence from the caregiver and a sense of its own identity while remaining securely connected. The child's efforts surround the dialectic between closeness and distance, separateness and connection. Blos (1967) wrote of the second process of individuation in adolescence as the young person negotiates the uncomfortable terrain of identity through separation and connection in a different way, this time leading to the solidification of a more adult sense of identity.

For Akhtar (1995) the journey of immigration may be likened to a third individuation—a developmental process akin to those earlier milestones in which the immigrant manages yet again the complex dynamics of separation and connection while seeking to establish their identity in still a new way. This is an apt and compelling metaphor inasmuch as the uncertainty of the immigration process can bring with it all the uncertainty about self and the world that is characteristic of those earlier times. Of course, all of this will take on a distinctive quality based on the personality of the individual, and whether that person is a child, adolescent, or adult. While children and adolescents are naturally in their initial phases of development to begin with, the process of immigration will still have an impact on the development of their identity and sense of self. Their experience of separation from a known environment and introduction to a foreign context with all that this entails must not be underestimated.

So how does this process of separation individuation manifest itself in the internal dynamics of the immigrant and the narrative he or she weaves from this experience? Not unlike the adolescent and even the young child in some ways, the process may call forth the use of splitting as a defense. Akhtar (1995) highlights the tendency of immigrants managing this process to alternately value and devalue both their country of origin and their new homeland. This may mean, for example, at times feeling nostalgic for and praising all that was wonderful back in their country while bemoaning all that is missing or flawed in the host country. At other times, the reverse may be true, when the immigrant feels a surge of pride or connection to their new land while decrying all that was terrible in their homeland and feeling grateful that they have left it all behind.

This pattern of valuing and devaluing is a balancing act of sorts in which the immigrant is searching for the best way to accommodate feelings of ambivalence toward both countries. From a narrative point of view, it involves a rehearsal of different versions of the story of the journey and the meaning this holds for the self. Which version will feel most true and most authentic? Which one fits with one's sense of self at least at that point in time? Like all narratives, these stories reflect the identity and perspective of the teller and may evolve over time.

Beyond the dynamics of splitting in the individual's view of their past and present homelands, these narratives can also involve an exploration of what the ideal balance of closeness and distance to the home country and culture may be (Akhtar, 1995). Is it better to hold on or let go or perhaps find some compromise in the middle? Similarly, the immigrant crafting and re-crafting this narrative will negotiate in an ongoing way their own self-representations in the context of their former life, present circumstances, and envisioned future. This involves establishing a balance between holding back—seeing oneself forever as a stranger in a foreign land, or propelling oneself toward total assimilation and the renunciation of the past self. Additionally, the immigrant may come to consider their new circumstances less from the point of view of a stranger examining the other from the outside, and more as a member or participant—a shift from second and third person (yours and theirs) to first person (mine and ours) (Akhtar, 1995). As we saw previously, language has very much to do with all this, since a change of dominant language in the environment not only serves to trigger the kind of separation we have been considering here, but also becomes an instrument in the reconfiguration of one's identity and sense of self (Mirsky, 1991).

Let me offer an example of some of these dynamics at play. Anika was 13 years old when her father brought her to see me. His initial description of the situation was that Anika had behavior problems at home. She was defiant and disrespectful. She didn't talk back or argue, but often coldly refused to comply with what she was asked to do. She also didn't offer her father the respect and deference he demanded according to their Indian culture and customs. Though the presenting problem seemed straightforward—at least from the father's point of view—I was confident that there would be more to the story. The fuller picture was actually quite a bit more complex.

Anika had come to live with her father in the United States only 3 months earlier, following the death of her mother in India. Anika had lived in India her whole life together with her mother and maternal grandmother. Her parents had divorced when she was an infant, and her father had moved to the United States where he found a job and settled down. He lived in an apartment with his new wife and their 8-year-old son, neither of whom Anika had met prior to her arrival in the States. When Anika's mother was diagnosed with cancer, her grandmother continued to provide stability; she had always been there. Anika told me that prior to her arrival several months before our meeting, she only recalled spending time with her father on two occasions when he had visited them in India while on vacation. There were intermittent phone calls, and presents on her birthday. Nonetheless, after her mother's death, the adults (including her father) decided that it was best for her to go live with him. By the time they told Anika about the plan, they had already bought the plane ticket. She traveled 2 weeks later.

Anika's first language was Hindi, but she spoke a good amount of English and we managed to communicate with only the occasional challenge. She presented as a shy and quiet girl. Though it was the fall, she came to her first session in a tiny pair of shorts, a gauzy white top, and sandals. She was quite apparently cold. When I asked her about it, she said that she didn't have any warm clothes and her stepmother was supposed to take her shopping that weekend. When her father was present in the session, he had a generally stern, frustrated demeanor to which Anika usually responded by lowering her gaze, folding her arms, and appearing to withdraw. When we were alone, she was more ready to engage, responding to inquiries about school, home life, the things she enjoyed, and of course all that she was missing of India, including her mother.

Consider what you understand from the story thus far. You are already beginning to tell yourself a story about Anika and her father too, perhaps the rest of the family as well. Anika is a young adolescent who only a few months earlier lost her mother after a prolonged battle with cancer. Even as she is mourning this profound loss, she is told that within 2 weeks she would leave the grandmother who was her main source of stability, her extended family, friends, school, and town—all that she had known complete with its sights, sounds, and smells—everything that was familiar to her. She would leave all that and travel to a place she had never seen, to live with a father she barely knew, along with a stepmother and half brother she had never met.

Anika's father was, in my estimation, a well-intentioned man trying to do what he thought was the right thing, to be the parent that he knew Anika needed, though he had never fulfilled that role in any meaningful way up to that point. The trouble was that he did not have the first clue about what Anika was really going through and had not been able to consider the story from her point of view. In his mind, Anika should be happy to be here. "Do you know how many young people would love to come to America?" he asked me. She should acknowledge what her father was doing and be grateful for it. But more than that, she should show him the respect and even affection that a good daughter owes her father.

That's where therapy came in. As happens often enough, Anika's father brought her to therapy seeking a solution to *her* problem, fixing *her* and getting *her* to behave appropriately. The course of treatment, though, took a different path. I began to work with Anika and her father, sometimes separately and sometimes together, from the point of view of competing, and in fact clashing, narratives. The first time I met with her father alone, I asked him to consider the story from Anika's perspective, and I laid out for him what I had heard explicitly and implicitly from her. He appeared genuinely sobered by this, realizing that he had missed the meaning of all these happenings for his daughter. He had been telling himself something of a hero story: a noble father who steps in and rescues his daughter when she most needs it. Whether or not you agree with the hero part of it, there is some truth to that story. He did step in; she did need him. But this was very different from the story Anika was telling, a story of loss on multiple levels, of confusion and disorientation, and even of some resentment. At a time when adolescents are trying mightily to figure out who they are, all of her points of references in the world had been taken away. Everything seemed up for grabs including her sense of self and what the future might look like. It was overwhelming.

Over the course of treatment we worked together on bridging the gaps between those vastly different narratives. Her father's increasing ability to listen to Anika's story and understand the events of the past months from her point of view was healing for her. There was no miracle, no tearful, melodramatic scene of father/daughter bonding. But they did draw closer. As her father and even her stepmother expressed more empathy for her and understood how overwhelmed she was, Anika was able to listen more to their story as well, and to see the ways they *were* trying to make things better. We talked about the loss of her mother and her mourning. We talked about the other things she felt she had lost in the course of this journey; there were more frequent phone calls back to India to help Anika feel an ongoing connection to what was familiar. We also talked about all the newness she seemed to encounter daily in this new place, and how it fit into the evolving story of her adjustment to a new life and a new sense of self.

All of this eased some tensions at home, at least to the point of what might be considered reasonable between a teenager and her parents. This was an important narrative component as well. I gently urged Anika's father, and even Anika herself, to resist the temptation to fantasize that their story together would go from one of conflict and resentment to one of storybook happiness. Even if they did not genuinely believe that this kind of fairytale ending would come, setting it up as the imagined goal of their narrative work would only make their real progress pale in comparison. My goal was to help them keep their real and developing relationship at the center of their story.

Narratives of Immigration Trauma

An important theme that we have touched on in some ways, but that I want to address in greater depth, concerns narratives of immigration trauma. In general, it is true to say that immigrants demonstrate remarkable patterns of resilience and health (The APA Presidential Task Force on Immigration, 2013). However, those working in the clinical arena must be ever attentive to the possible presence of trauma, assessing our immigrant clients sensitively and carefully (Fortuna et al., 2008). This means being open to the way clients from different cultures may express their distress (Nichter, 1981). As Herman (1992) commented, "Psychological trauma is an affliction of the powerless (p. 33)." Permeating the immigration narrative for many of our clients may be experiences of politically inspired violence or conditions of social unrest and lawlessness (this includes the witnessing of violence), sexual assault, domestic violence, torture, unsanitary or otherwise substandard living conditions, and exposure to exploitation (Foster, 2001; Levers & Hyatt-Burkhart, 2012). These may be found in the country of origin from which the immigrant is fleeing, often at even greater risk to themselves and their families, as well as throughout the experience of transit, or upon arrival at their destination.

It has been estimated that up to 54% of immigrants in clinical examples have been exposed to political violence, and this is often not disclosed to healthcare providers (Eisenman, Gelberg, Liu, & Shapiro, 2003). Though exposure to such potentially traumatogenic circumstances can result in post-traumatic stress disorder, anxiety, depression, disordered substance use, and interpersonal problems such as domestic violence, mental health care is generally underutilized for those who have been exposed to psychosocial trauma (Levers & Hyatt-Burkhart, 2012; Rasmussen, Rosenfeld, Reeves, & Keller, 2007). Fortuna et al. (2008) outline a number of barriers that may exist for immigrants who need to access such services. These include "language, insurance, economic barriers, and documentation status" (p. 437) as well as issues such as shame, stigma, reliance on family and community for assistance, and becoming so accustomed to things like political violence that it does not seem like a reason to seek care. This last observation reminds us that, in the end, the nature of trauma is always dependent on the subjective appraisal of the experience by the one exposed to it (Rasmussen et al., 2007).

Politics, Culture, and the Immigration Narrative

The social, cultural, and political debate about immigration and what it means has moved to the forefront of the national and even global conversation. Since the beginning of the 2016 US Presidential race, and in forums ranging from scholarly policy analyses of refugee and humanitarian crises to television and print journalism, to social media, to dinner-table conversations around the nation, we have been listening to diverse perspectives and competing narratives. According to Edwards and Herder (2012), social and cultural attitudes in the United States about immigration have always involved a dialectic between what they identify as themes of inclusion and exclusion. In our social discourse, immigrants have been identified as among our greatest resources, grounded in the history of immigration that led to the founding of the nation. At other times, immigration has been painted as a threat to our way of life, and a drain on our resources. The authors note that this history can be seen running through the rhetoric of US Presidents on the topic. Some Presidents have highlighted one or the other, while others such as George W. Bush have tried to strike a balance between the two (Edwards & Herder, 2012).

On June 16, 2015, Donald Trump announced his campaign for the Presidency of the United States, and the theme of immigration was front and center. Media outlets across the political spectrum covered the speech and took note, whether in agreement or disagreement, of the rhetoric contained in the speech. Trump declared[1] that the United States is in "serious trouble" and that "We don't have victories anymore." He added, "The U.S. has become a dumping ground for everybody else's problems." This led into what was perhaps the most often cited and replayed portion of the speech. "When Mexico sends its people, they're not sending their best. They're not sending you. They're not sending you. [Pointing to individuals in the crowd.] They're sending people that have lots of problems, and they're bringing those problems with us [sic]. They're bringing drugs. They're bringing crime. They're rapists. And some, I assume, are good people."

From a narrative point of view and mindful of our professional commitment to social justice (National Association of Social Workers, 2008), we might examine the nature of the rhetorical devices used here and their impact on the formation of public perception. Stewart (2012) has studied the way in which narrative has been used to accomplish a wide range of goals including winning elections and bringing about social change. She writes that "in politics, narratives are purposeful and strategic," and that they "produce winners and losers" (p. 594). How is this accomplished?

---

[1] The full text of Donald Trump's campaign launch speech may be found at http://time.com/3923128/donald-trump-announcement-speech/. Passages quoted here are taken from this source.

Stewart turns for insight to the work of Smith (2005) who delineated a four-part typology of narratives to examine how countries decide to wage war. He refers to them as the lower mimetic, tragic, romantic, and apocalyptic. For our purposes, the two that are most significant are the lower mimetic and the apocalyptic. According to Smith, the lower mimetic approach is the most straightforward inasmuch as it is driven by facts and is based on an analysis that is pragmatic and reasoned. It also tends to be the least inspiring or emotionally appealing. The apocalyptic narrative, on the other hand, frames its story in emotionally provocative terms in order to elicit an affective response from readers or listeners. This is the kind of narrative that we know has extraordinary power to set political and social causes in motion (Polletta, 2006).

Stewart's (2012) position that this same rhetorical contest is at play in discussions of immigration could perhaps be applied to Trump's campaign launch address as an example of apocalyptic narrative. This kind of speech makes use of master tropes and literary devices such as metaphor, and synecdoche wherein singular examples or statistical exceptions are presented as the rule (Stewart, 2012). Borrowing Smith's terminology, this apocalyptic style narrative is effective in some quarters because it taps into the deep well of collective fear that has gripped society in the face of terrorism. This strategy of responding to legitimate concerns about public safety by projecting fantasies of badness onto a generalized other is consistent with the thinking of both Volkan (1988) and Moskowitz (1995) that we have reviewed. This form of splitting on cultural and even global levels serves to set us apart from and blame the other as a whole.

It should also be noted that in an effort to counter this trend, progressive media and popular culture may unwittingly reinforce some of the same myths they seek to dispel. Sowards and Pineda (2013) have analyzed the portrayal of immigrant narratives in contemporary media and suggest that in trying to personalize the experience of immigrants (e.g., by featuring individual immigrant stories) as a way of generating empathy, they may have in fact reinforced negative stereotypes. For example, just as an anti-immigrant rhetoric might rely on the use of a carefully chosen example of an immigrant committing a horrific crime as a way of inciting a distrust of immigrants as a group, so too the selective highlighting of an extraordinary story of immigrant virtue and success may leave listeners and viewers wondering why "they can't all be like that." This, in turn, reinforces the naïve expectation that, despite whatever obstacles they may face, immigrants and other poor and marginalized groups could be successful if they were only willing to work hard enough and pull themselves up by their bootstraps.

As social workers and clinicians, it is our responsibility to be thoughtful and sophisticated participants in the political process, reading and listening with a critical eye and ear for the ways in which narratives are being crafted and the purposes they are intended to serve. Particularly if we intend to work with group such as immigrants that have so long and so easily been marginalized and disenfranchised, and that have so commonly been seen as dispensable or not seen at all, such that they can fall victim to the traumas inflicted by self-interested powers, then we must learn not only to hear and call out narratives of oppression. We must join with these communities in crafting narratives of healing and liberation.

Case Example

Diana came to the agency seeking help because she was having difficulty sleeping. She was in her early 40s and lived with her three young daughters in an apartment in the neighborhood, having come to the United States 5 years earlier from the Balkans where she was born and raised. She had several extended family members in the area. She worked second shift at a local factory. A thorough assessment revealed that Diana was suffering from post-traumatic stress disorder. Though it was her distress over a lack of sleep that brought her in, Diana also endorsed flashbacks, nightmares, an exaggerated startle response, feelings of irritability and avoidance, and increasing isolation from friends and family. More and more she relied on her daughters to manage affairs in the world while she confined herself largely to her bedroom, or at least the apartment.

The story behind Diana's PTSD symptoms was difficult for her to tell, and I could see that she was mustering the courage to do so. She presented as agitated, but it was subtle, like a vibration just under the surface that you can feel even though it is hard to see on the outside. She spoke quite quickly, almost a staccato rhythm that came in short bursts, followed by long runs when she would run out of air and have to catch her breath. Diana told me that 6 years previously, her husband had been murdered in their town. He was a lawyer for the government and had been working on investigating and prosecuting leaders of a major drug trafficking ring. One day, as he was leaving court, he was gunned down as he descended the courthouse steps. Diana told me that she lived only a couple of blocks away, and when a neighbor said that there had been gunfire at the courthouse, she ran down there to find her husband lying on the steps, riddled with bullets from machine gun fire. He was already dead. The men who killed him were long gone, and as was usually the case when these kinds of things happened, no one saw a thing.

Diana was distraught. Though she and her husband had been having some difficulties (he has moved temporarily to his mother's house several months before), he was still her husband and she loved him. He came by the house every day, usually before or after work and sometimes both. He spent time with Diana and the girls. He often stayed for dinner. They were working it out. But there she was, screaming, crying, practically laying on the courthouse steps holding her husband's body in her arms. A small crowd formed but just stared at her—faces blank—knowing but never daring to speak. She heard the sound of approaching sirens.

This was the scene Diana said haunted her—one she had replayed in nightmares and flashbacks countless times, leaving her shaken, nauseous, and sometimes gasping for air. At times, she told me, her daughters would startle her out of her trance claiming that they had been talking to her. Didn't she hear what they said? No. She didn't. Her husband's death was the last in a long line of traumas they had experienced. There were threatening notes and packages that arrived in the mail. Once there were two men with guns who pushed their way into the house when she answered the door. Only Diana and her daughters were home. After rifling the house, they left a message for her husband, "Watch your back." There were other things too. The news always had stories about escalations in violence between the drug traffickers and the police. But there were also plenty of accusations of corruption among police and government officials who had been paid off to turn a blind eye and not disrupt the extremely lucrative drug trade. There was infighting among the traffickers that sometimes erupted on the streets. The sound of gunshots whether near or far was common enough. The previous year there had been a car bomb about half a mile away. The sight of men with machine guns and other arms was familiar. Diana always had the same advice for her daughters. Though she rarely let them go outside alone, she told them, "Always give them a wide berth. If possible walk the other way, but don't make it obvious. And don't make eye contact. Don't run; but don't linger either."

Diana recalled one morning when she had to show her daughters exactly what she meant. As she was walking them to school, they turned a corner only to find the dead body of a young man lying by the curb. He had been shot in the head. They knew him. He was a young man from the neighborhood, barely more than a boy really. He was friendly, and nice. And, they learned, he had been working as a courier for one of the trafficking rings. When they saw his body, Diana said, the girls began to cry and repeat, "Mommy, mommy, look! Look who it is, Mommy! We know him!" "No!" Diana said. "We don't know him. We don't know anything. Keep walking! Don't look and keep walking!" They walked right past the dead body and she dropped them off at school. Diana returned home by a different route. Diana said, "You know, as we passed by, I could see them out of the corner of my eye. These men stood across the street, guns draped on their shoulders, stone faced. They just stared down everyone who walked past. Everyone knew the truth; they had killed him. But what did they care? No one could touch them and they knew it."

All of this was enough to make Diana live with a nearly constant sense of dread, but when her husband was assassinated, as she put it, she knew that was the end. They had to go. There was no one to keep them safe now. It took some time to arrange, time when they rarely left the house unless they had to, but eventually they were able to come to the United States. They settled in New Jersey because it was where they had some family. Diana hoped that she had put enough distance between her and the past that they could start a new life and be safe. But the memories would not let her be.

Diana and I worked on several fronts. The first involved helping her to develop some healthy and effective coping strategies so she could manage better her feelings of hyperarousal and tension. This enabled us to work with the often-fragmented parts of the narrative of her trauma. The pieces of the story were often confusing to me, and to Diana herself for that matter. However, with time and patience, Diana was increasingly able to put some order to her narrative (Schauer, Neuner, & Elbert, 2011). As she did so, her ability to self-regulate improved, and her symptoms began to subside a bit. This measure of progress helped Diana have the courage to continue our work.

To the extent of her tolerance, we also worked on understanding the meaning she made of all that had happened to her and her family. In the beginning of course, all the interpretations of which she was aware had a negative valence. They involved how corrupt and untrustworthy people are, and how those who try to do the right thing will only get punished in the end. Therapeutically, it was important to be able to sit with these meanings of her experience and not contradict them. An impulse that can arise in this kind of work and that must be resisted is to want the client to move more quickly than they are able to a more peaceful emotional place. Though therapists want this for the client, it often has more to do with their own discomfort and the difficulty of containing emotions and a narrative that can feel so toxic. But containment is precisely what is called for.

Over some time, and as her confidence in my understanding and empathy grew, Diana and I could explore some other meanings. Diana was able to remind herself that her husband was a good man who made extraordinary sacrifices in the service of what he knew to be right. She was able to tell me the story of people, both at home and in the United States, who had shown themselves to be honest and true in many ways, people she knew she could count on. Diana was also able to begin telling something of a different story about herself. In keeping with what we know about the phenomenon of posttraumatic growth (Calhoun & Tedeschi, 2006; Meichenbaum, 2006; Neimeyer, 2004, 2006; Tedeschi & Calhoun, 2004), Diana was able to identify ways in which she had surprised herself, and her daughters had surprised her as well. She was able to tell me about her own toughness and inner resolve in the face of such frightening circumstances. She told me a story of a mother's determination to protect her children in the face of danger, taking on challenges she never thought she could handle alone, coming to a new country, and building a life, all in order to keep them safe and promise them a future, just as their husband and father would have wanted for them. She recounted the remarkable signs of resilience in her daughters and the ways they were thriving in their new situation.

The third front on which we worked related to Diana's adjustment to her life in the United States. She struggled in many of the ways we have discussed in this chapter to make sense of all the newness that surrounded her. She lived in a largely ethnic community, so while she faced occasional challenges with English, they were not a great obstacle in her day-to-day life. She was confused by customs and systems that Americans seemed to take for granted. One of these was the healthcare system. Without health insurance, Diana made use of a local hospital's clinic. Difficulties getting an appointment, long waits, crowds, and as she described it never being seen by the same doctor twice were hard to get used to. To be sure, native-born Americans who used the clinic had to deal with the same conditions. But it all had a distinctly foreign character to Diana that made it difficult to understand.

Given her background, Diana also had a great deal of difficulty trusting people who were in supposed position of authority. In her narrative, there was so much corruption in the world that powerful people were never to be trusted. Each of them was in it for their own gain and would not give a second thought about what it meant to someone like her. This came into play, for example, when she went to a clinic appointment to talk with the doctor about the results of some blood work she had done. Following a previous appointment when the resident she saw ordered the blood work, she was only able to be seen in the lab a month later. When she called the clinic to schedule a follow-up, they gave her an appointment 3 months later. On the day of that appointment, a new resident came into the exam room and asked her to explain why she was there. She told him about the blood work that had been done and explained she was there to follow up about the results. When the resident looked at the paper work, he said with clear frustration that since they were 3 months old, they were perfectly useless. He told her to have the blood work done again and then come back. He turned and left the room. Diana was furious.

Though she managed to find a sympathetic clerk who tried to arrange for timely appointments, Diana came to session telling me that everyone in the clinic was corrupt and that it was all a scam. This was just another example of the powerful walking all over the poor, and in this case trying to make money off their illness and suffering. Though I certainly shared in Diana's indignation about the injustice of such a flawed system of health care for the poor, and I let her know it, for Diana there was something more in it. For her, it was personal. It tapped into her past experiences in a way that made her feel angry, and exploited, and even a bit paranoid.

Another system that evoked difficult feelings for Diana was the educational system. In her native country, she and her husband paid for their daughters to attend a fine private school. Now, in her inner-city neighborhood in New Jersey, they attended the local public school. Diana sensed that it was inadequate in many ways, but felt powerless to do anything about it. This was frustrating for her. Nonetheless, her girls did well in school and the teachers had positive things to say about them. Diana came to session one day and told me that her eldest daughter, a senior in high school, said that she would like to apply to a local state university to become a nurse. Her daughter was very bright and Diana was proud of her. The university she was thinking of was known for their nursing program, and the guidance counselor at the high school was sure that she would get in.

Diana told her daughter that, while she was very proud of her, she thought applying to university would be a big mistake. Diana said that her daughter looked shocked and deflated all at once and that she began to cry. I asked Diana what made her feel that it was a bad idea. "Look," she said, "I'm sure my daughter would be a wonderful nurse. But we don't have that kind of money. The only way she could do that would be to hope for financial aid and to take out loans. And I told her, that's a big mistake. Taking out loans with the government means you have to give them all this information about you. Then they own you! It's just a trick to put people in debt for the rest of their lives. You can't trust these people. You should see all the paperwork the school sent home, and all the information you have to turn over to them. No. I told my daughter that the better way would be to go to that school downtown that offers the home health aid program. We could afford that and it's only a couple of months. Then she could start bringing some money into the house too. She can start saving, and when she has enough saved to go to university and become a nurse, then she can go. And she won't have to answer any questions or owe anything to the government."

I listened patiently to Diana and could see how upsetting the issue was to her. She hated disappointing her daughter, but thought she was young and naïve and didn't understand the way the world worked. Again, Diana was deeply mistrustful of government, large systems, and people in authority. This issue brought them all together for her, and threw their financial life in as well. As we discussed it, it turned out that Diana found the higher education system in the United States very confusing. Why did it cost so much money? Why did they make you take courses that had nothing to do with the career you wanted? Wasn't it all just a scam? I explained to her that there were probably a lot of Americans who would ask the same questions and who were also confused by the system. She chuckled and relaxed a bit. We talked about it more and compared the salary of a home health aid with that of a registered nurse. She did not realize how much a nurse could earn. We also talked about the feasibility of saving enough money to pay for 4 years of university out of pocket. She said that the guidance counselor told her daughter that applying for financial aid and taking out loans was very common, and asked me if that was true. I said it was. She then added that the guidance counselor also said that because of her high GPA, Diana's daughter would likely qualify for a scholarship. I asked Diana what she made of all that. She said she would think about it.

Still, the road was not without obstacles and pitfalls, and an immigration narrative like Diana's will rarely evolve on an uninterrupted path toward integration and health. One day Diana came to session and it was clear that she was quite agitated. She spoke quickly and in fragments. I first helped Diana calm herself and then asked her to tell me what happened. She had gone to her corner store that morning to get a newspaper, just as she did most days. She had become somewhat friendly with the storeowner and they were on a first-name basis. He was from her country as well, and they had spoken casually about the towns where they were born and had lived. But he knew nothing else about her. Diana was very private.

The storeowner told her that morning that something odd had happened. A well-dressed man came into the store. He was clearly from their country and spoke in their native language. The owner had never seen him before and it was evident that the man did not live in the neighborhood. He was probably just visiting or was newly arrived. The man ordered a cup of coffee and told the owner that he was trying to find a friend. He named Diana—first and last names. He also named the town where Diana had come from—the town where her husband had been killed. He had heard that Diana lived in the neighborhood. He asked the storeowner if he knew Diana and exactly where she lived. The storeowner told Diana that something seemed suspicious about him. If they were really friends why would he arrive in the neighborhood and have to ask where Diana lived? He told the man he wasn't sure if he knew anyone by that name. So many people come and go and he usually knows them only by face, not name. Besides, he certainly wouldn't know where she lived.

The man pressed further. If the owner did know Diana or someone who might be her, did he have any idea where she worked? What time of day did she usually come into the store? The owner offered no information. He asked the man his name and if he wanted to leave a phone number. That was all right, he said. He would just ask around to find his friend. Then he left. The owner said that he went to the window and saw the stranger get into a car where another man was waiting.

Diana was near panic, convinced that members of the drug trafficking ring had found her. She had tried so hard to disappear, to leave the past behind. But now they were here and they were looking for her. I have to admit that the situation was odd and Diana's reaction had me somewhat anxious as well. On the one hand it sounded like the stuff of movies. On the other hand, how could she safely be sure what was going on? I asked Diana if she thought there was any chance that someone, a friend from her hometown, had come to New Jersey and was trying to connect with her. She said no. She had thought of it, trying to remain calm and not jump to conclusions.

Earlier in the day, before our session, she had called home. She spoke to her mother and one of her sisters. Had anyone from the town spoken to them? Had anyone asked about her? They said no. She asked if they had told anyone, even in casual conversation, where she had gone to live. Both her mother and her sister said that it had never come up. It was not so unusual for people from the town to move away. Besides, Diana had always been one to keep to herself. The only ones likely to be interested were close friends, and they already knew. What's more, everyone in their inner circle was aware of what really happened to Diana's husband and the way the drug traffickers operated. No one would dare say a thing.

As I sat with Diana I found myself wishing that I could find a perfectly rational explanation for what had happened that day. In my mind, it could be perfectly innocent. And I had no way of knowing, nor did she. That was the problem. Diana was able to accept support and, when she was calm, see that there was no certainty in her conclusion about the stranger. Still, she felt like she needed to be cautious and I told her that I agreed it was probably wise. She did have a few friends in the neighborhood and some extended family. She would ask everyone to be attentive. Even the owner of the corner store knew instinctively to refrain from giving out information. Diana gave him her phone number and he agreed to call right away if the man came around again. We talked about whether to go to the police, but she felt that she had nothing substantial enough to tell them. What could they do?

In the end, the strange man never did come around again. Diana remained cautious for herself and her daughters. She was aware that there were people she could turn to for help, and though she wound up not needing it in this situation, it was good for her to know that friends and family cared and were there to support them.

Diana and I continued to work on our various fronts—healing the narratives of the past, and building her story of the present and future. Increasingly, as we worked through and integrated much of the pain and loss of her past, we were able to focus more on the here and now and on what she wanted for her life going forward. She continued to struggle at times and she had some challenging days. Her narrative of mistrust was triggered over and over again by the struggles of daily living. At those times, we would refocus on the narrative of success and growth. That helped her. She did decide to let her daughter apply to university. She was accepted of course, with a large scholarship and a small loan. Her other daughters were thriving as well, and we used their growth to strengthen Diana's own story of success. Her symptoms of PTSD were better contained and she was developing a new sense of herself as a strong woman and a strong mother in a new land.

Questions and Activities for Discussion and Further Reflection

1. What do you know of the immigration story of your own family? There is almost certainly a story to be told. If you are not sure, or have never heard about it, talk with some of your family's elders. What common elements of immigration narratives are part of your story? What stands out to you as unique?
2. Discuss as a class the social work values that come into play in our work with immigrant individuals, families, and communities? Consult the Code of Ethics as a guide.
3. Visit the websites for the Pew Center and for the U.N. High Commission on Refugees. Both have a wealth of statistics and reports on the status of immigrants and refugees in the United States and around the world. Take some time to read and examine them. Share what you learned, particularly anything that surprised you, with a friend, family, or your class. How does the information you find there compare to the narratives you hear coming from the culture?
4. In a similar vein, go to the website and review the work of Human Rights Watch, Amnesty International, or another human rights organization. What are they doing to raise awareness and enhance human rights around the world (including in the United States)?
5. Do you work with immigrant clients? Do you know about their experience of the immigration journey? If so, what themes in their story are similar to those discussed in the chapter? What differences do you hear? If you do not know their immigration story, talk with your supervisor about the possibility of exploring it if pertinent.
6. Have you ever been in a different cultural context where you did not fully understand what was happening around you or what was expected of you? Have you ever been in a place where you could not speak the language? Reflect on what that experience was like for you. Consider all the components of your own history, culture(s), and social environment, not just the obvious ones. If you were compelled to move to a different country, what losses would you sustain? What would you miss most? How do you think you might cope with that loss? Consider brainstorming with your class or sharing your own reflections.
7. Go back to the variety of case illustrations throughout the chapter or the case of Diana at the end. What stood out to you most about immigration narratives from those stories? Did one in particular strike you more than the others? Perhaps you imagine that one of those clients might be easier or more challenging to work with? What makes that so for you? Consider role-playing the case with a peer. See what it might be like to sit with that person's story and then work with them from a narrative point of view.
8. Tune into current and developing political speech about immigration. Pay attention to speeches that are given. If you can't watch them live, find a video or a transcript. Read news articles in print or online about immigration. Identify the narrative that is being told about immigration and critique it. What do you hear? What don't you hear? Now try to find a piece that features an opposing view. Be attentive to the way the argument is made and what the speakers or

writers draw on in making their case. What do you think about their positions? (This exercise can be done individually or as a class. It can also be used to reflect on a number of other social, cultural, and political issues).

References

Ainslie, R. C., Tummala-Narra, P., Harlem, A., Barbanel, L., & Ruth, R. (2013). Contemporary psychoanalytic views on the experience of immigration. *Psychoanalytic Psychology, 30*(4), 663–679. https://doi.org/10.1037/a0034588

Akhtar, S. (1995). A third individuation: Immigration, identity, and the psychoanalytic process. *Journal of the American Psychoanalytic Association, 43*(4), 1051–1084. https://doi.org/10.1177/000306519504300406

Alessi, E. J. (2016). Resilience in sexual and gender minority forced migrants: A qualitative analysis. *Traumatology, 22*, 203–213.

Arbona, C., Olvera, N., Rodriguez, N., Hagan, J., Linares, A., & Wiesner, M. (2010). Acculturative stress among documented and undocumented Latino immigrants in the United States. *Hispanic Journal of Behavioral Sciences, 32*(3), 362–384.

Azarian-Ceccato, N. (2010). Reverberations of the Armenian genocide: Narrative's intergenerational transmission and the task of not forgetting. *Narrative Inquiry, 20*(1), 106–123. https://doi.org/10.1075/ni.20.1.06aza

Benish-Weisman, M. (2009). Between trauma and redemption: Story form differences in immigrant narratives of successful and nonsuccessful immigration. *Journal of Cross Cultural Psychology, 40*(6), 953–968.

Blos, P. (1967). The second individuation process of adolescence. *Psychoanalytic Study of the Child, 22*, 162–186.

Bruner, J. (1986). *Actual minds, possible worlds*. Cambridge, MA: Harvard University Press.

Bruner, J. (1990). *Acts of meaning*. Cambridge, MA: Harvard University Press.

Bruner, J. (1991). The narrative construction of reality. *Critical Inquiry, 18*(1), 1–21.

Calhoun, L. G., & Tedeschi, R. G. (Eds.). (2006). *Handbook of posttraumatic growth: Research and practice*. New York: Lawrence Erlbaum Associates.

Dion, K. K., & Dion, K. L. (2001). Gender and cultural adaptations in immigrant families. *Journal of Social Issues, 57*(3), 511–521.

Edwards, J. A., & Herder, R. (2012). Melding a new immigration narrative? President George W. Bush and the immigration debate. *Howard Journal of Communications, 23*(1), 40–65. https://doi.org/10.1080/10646175.2012.641878

Eisenman, D. P., Gelberg, L., Liu, H., & Shapiro, M. F. (2003). Mental health and health-related quality of life among adult Latino primary care patient living in the United States with previous exposure to political violence. *Journal of the American Medical Association, 290*(5), 627–634.

Fortuna, L. R., Porche, M. V., & Alegria, M. (2008). Political violence, psychosocial trauma, and the context of mental health services use among immigrant Latinos in the United States. *Ethnicity and Health, 13*(5), 435–463.

Foster, R. P. (2001). When immigration is trauma: Guidelines for the individual and family clinician. *American Journal of Orthopsychiatry, 71*(2), 153–170. https://doi.org/10.1037/0002-9432.71.2.153

Gergen, K. J., & Gergen, M. M. (1988). Narrative and the self as relationship. In L. Berkowits (Ed.), *Advances in experimental social psychology* (Vol. 21, pp. 17–54). San Diego, CA: Academic Press.

Grim, B. J., & Finke, R. (2011). *The price of freedom denied: Religious persecution and conflict in the twenty-first century*. New York: Cambridge University Press.

Hall, E. T. (1963). A system for the notation of proxemic behavior. *American Anthropologist, 65*(5), 1003–1026. https://doi.org/10.1525/aa.1963.65.5.02a00020

Herman, J. (1992). *Trauma and recovery*. New York: Basic Books.

Hollander, N. C. (2006). Negotiating trauma and loss in the migration experience: Roundtable on global woman. *Studies in Gender and Sexuality, 7*(1), 61–70.

Kidder, T. (2010). *Strength in what remains*. New York: Random House.

Levers, L. L., & Hyatt-Burkhart, D. (2012). Immigration reform and the potential for psychosocial trauma: The missing link of lived human experience. *Analyses of Social Issues and Public Policy (ASAP), 12*(1), 68–77. https://doi.org/10.1111/j.1530-2415.2011.01254.x

Lindsey, L. L. (2015). *Gender roles: A sociological perspective* (6th ed.). New York: Routledge.

Lopez, G., & Bialik, K. (2017). Key findings about U.S. immigration, 1–14. Retrieved from Pew Research Center. http://www.pewresearch.org/fact-tank/2017/05/03/key-findings-about-u-s-immigrants/

Mahler, M. S. (1963). Thoughts and development and individuation. *Psychoanalytic Study of the Child, 81*, 307–324.

Mahler, M. S., Pine, F., & Bergman, A. (1975). *The psychological birth of the human infant*. New York: Basic Books.

Matsumoto, D. (2006). Culture and nonverbal behavior. In V. Manusov & M. L. Patterson (Eds.), *The SAGE handbook of nonverbal communication* (pp. 219–236). Thousand Oaks, CA: Sage Publications.

Meichenbaum, D. (2006). Resilience and posttraumatic growth. In L. G. Calhoun & R. G. Tedeschi (Eds.), *Handbook of posttraumatic growth: Research and practice* (pp. 355–367). New York: Lawrence Erlbaum Associates.

Mirsky, J. (1991). Language in migration: Separation individuation conflicts in relation to the mother tongue and the new language. *Psychotherapy: Theory, Research, Practice, Training, 28*(4), 618–624. https://doi.org/10.1037/0033-3204.28.4.618

Moskowitz, M. (1995). Ethnicity and the fantasy of ethnicity. *Psychoanalytic Psychology, 12*(4), 547–555. https://doi.org/10.1037/h0079690

National Association of Social Workers. (2008). *The NASW code of ethics*. Washington, DC: NASW Press.

Neimeyer, R. A. (2004). Fostering posttraumatic growth: A narrative contribution. *Psychological Inquiry, 15*, 53–59.

Neimeyer, R. A. (2006). Re-storying loss: Fostering growth in the posttraumatic narrative. In L. G. Calhoun & R. G. Tedeschi (Eds.), *Handbook of posttraumatic growth: Research and practice* (pp. 68–80). New York: Lawrence Erlbaum Associates.

Nichter, M. (1981). Idioms of distress: Alternatives in the expression of psychosocial distress: A case study from South India. *Culture, Medicine and Psychiatry, 5*(4), 379–408.

Nieri, T., Grindal, M., Adams, M. A., Cookston, J. T., Fabricius, W. V., Parke, R. D., & Saenz, D. S. (2016). Reconsidering the "acculturation gap" narrative through the analysis of parent-adolescent acculturation differences in Mexican American families. *Journal of Family Issues, 37*(14), 1919–1944.

Polletta, F. (2006). *It was like a fever: Storytelling in protest and politics*. Chicago, IL: University of Chicago Press.

Portman, S., & Weyl, D. (2013). LGBT refugee resettlement in the US: Emerging best practices. *Forced Migration Review, 42*, 44–47.

Rasmussen, A., Rosenfeld, B., Reeves, K., & Keller, A. S. (2007). The subjective experience of trauma and subsequent PTSD in a sample of undocumented immigrants. *The Journal of Nervous and Mental Disease, 195*(2), 137–143.

Schauer, M., Neuner, F., & Elbert, T. (2011). *Narrative exposure therapy: A short-term treatment for traumatic stress disorders*. Cambridge, MA: Hogrefe.

Smith, P. (2005). *Why war? The cultural logic of Iraq, the Gulf War, and Suez*. Chicago, IL: University of Chicago Press.

Sowards, S. K., & Pineda, R. D. (2013). Immigrant narratives and popular culture in the United States: Border spectacle, unmotivated sympathies, and individualized responsibilities. *Western Journal of Communication, 77*(1), 72–91. https://doi.org/10.1080/10570314.2012.693648

Spence, D. P. (1982). *Narrative truth and historical truth.* New York: W.W. Norton.

Stewart, J. (2012). Fiction over facts: How competing narrative forms explain policy in a new immigration destination. *Sociological Forum, 27*(3), 591–616. https://doi.org/10.1111/j.1573-7861.2012.01337.x

Tedeschi, R. G., & Calhoun, L. G. (2004). Posttraumatic growth: Conceptual foundations and empirical evidence. *Psychological Inquiry, 15,* 1–18.

The APA Presidential Task Force on Immigration. (2013). Crossroads: The psychology of immigration in the new century. *Journal of Latina/o Psychology, 1*(3), 133–148. https://doi.org/10.1037/lat0000001

Tummala-Narra, P. (2014). Cultural identity in the context of trauma and immigration from a psychoanalytic perspective. *Psychoanalytic Psychology, 31*(3), 396–409. https://doi.org/10.1037/a0036539

U.S. Citizenship and Immigration Services. (2015). Refugees & asylum. Retrieved from https://www.uscis.gov/humanitarian/refugees-asylum

United Nations High Commission on Refugees. (2017). Figures at a glance. Retrieved from http://www.unhcr.org/en-us/figures-at-a-glance.html?query=how many refugees are there in the world?

Viruell-Fuentes, E. A., Miranda, P. Y., & Abdulrahim, S. (2012). More than culture: Structural racism, intersectionality theory, and immigrant health. *Social Science & Medicine, 75*(12), 2099–2106. https://doi.org/10.1016/j.socscimed.2011.12.037

Volkan, V. (1988). *The need to have enemies and allies: From clinical practice to international relationships.* New York: Jason Aronson.

Volkan, V. (2007). Not letting go: From individual perennial mourners to societies with entitlement ideologies. In L. G. Fioroni, S. Loewkowicz, & T. Bokanowski (Eds.), *On Freud's "mourning and melancholia"* (pp. 90–109). London: International Psychoanalytic Association.

Chapter 7
Moving on: Narrative Perspectives on Grief and Loss

Guiding Questions

How has the shared story of the nature and meaning of grief and loss evolved over time? How do we understand the dynamics of grief and loss now?
What does narrative have to tell us about the experience of grief and loss on personal, familial, and social levels?
What are the dynamics involved in the process of renegotiating a sense of meaning following a significant loss?
What are the varieties of loss that we may encounter in our own lives as well as in the lives of our clients?
For clinicians, what is the nature of grief work from a narrative point of view? How might we engage in that work sensitively with our clients?

It is a part of every human life—every human story. Grief and loss touch us all in some way, at some point in time. If you have been spared their pain up to this point, the thought of it might still evoke some feelings of dread. You might just as soon push the thought of it to the side, somewhere out of your consciousness. You know it will come eventually. For some of us, it may feel as though our story is punctuated by losses that usher us into the darkness of grief and bereavement, and most of the time to the other side. Narratively speaking, this is a place of renegotiation, of forging something new of our selves and of the world. But there may scarcely be a part of the common human experience that is so often feared, renounced, hurried through, buried, or otherwise rejected as the alternating tumult and void of grief.

For us as social workers and therapists, the clinical space brings us all the time, even without our conscious awareness, to the question of how similar a client's experience is to our own. Because we are human, and if we are paying attention, we can often find those points of comparison that, if we are skilled and remain disciplined, we almost certainly keep to ourselves, though we may use them sometimes with greater or lesser success. Yes, everyone's experience is unique in its particulars, but it is the shared layers of our stories that are the roots of empathy. This may be truer of nothing more than it is of grief and loss. Whether it relates to the finality of death, our own or that of another, or to a different type of loss that may be no less painful, we are all given a portion of grief in this life.

There are, in fact, so many varieties of grief and loss that it would not be possible to recount them all and do them justice in the space of this chapter. So my hope is this: that we will explore together the major narrative components and dynamics of grief that we need to be aware of as clinicians, as well as an overview of the kinds of grief and loss with which we are invited to sit in our work. By doing so, I hope that we will be better prepared to walk with another through an uncertain terrain that is at once so shared and yet so deeply personal.

Let's begin with the observation that we can speak of a narrative understanding of grief and loss on at least two levels. There is the storied nature of the ways loss has touched our lives directly or indirectly. We will turn our attention to this shortly. But there is also the narrative that we have woven about grief and loss themselves, the story we tell about their nature and their dynamics. How are we to wrap our minds around grief and loss and the impact they may have in our lives? This is, without exaggeration, a story that we have perhaps been exploring since the beginnings of human consciousness. It is treated in the scriptural texts of all the major religious traditions. It has been a significant theme throughout the history of literature and other forms of artistic expression, as well as philosophy and science.

For our purposes, let's begin somewhat closer to home. From a social science perspective, Neimeyer and Harris (2016) offer a concise review of the major schools of thought regarding bereavement ("the condition of having lost a significant other or attachment figure" p. 163) and grief (the distress caused by this loss) over the past century. Freud's (1917/1957) effort to explore the nature and presentation of grief as well as to offer an understanding of its dynamics that would be useful in the clinical situation has been perhaps the most widely influential of all. Freud distinguishes between mourning (grief associated with loss) and melancholia (what we would refer to as depression). This distinction foreshadows reflection on what we more currently think of as the relationship between "normal" and "complicated" grief, the latter referring to "grieving that fails to move forward adaptively as the person integrates the loss, instead remaining intense, preoccupying, prolonged, and life-limiting" (Neimeyer & Harris, 2016, p. 163). The heart of the matter, for Freud, pertains to what he refers to as *decathexis*—the withdrawal of the psychic energy that one has invested in the lost object (person) such that this energy is available again for the ongoing living of the bereaved. Decathexis, for Freud, results in the normal resolution of the process of grieving. The inability to decathect, however, results in melancholia.

The next major shift in thinking about grief and loss came with the emergence of stage theory. As the name suggests, stage theory conceptualizes grief as proceeding in a predictable, stepwise fashion that is seen as more or less universally applicable. The most well-known example of this approach is the work of Elizabeth Kubler-Ross (1969), a psychiatrist who presented a model of grief as evolving through five stages: denial, anger, bargaining, depression, and acceptance. Kubler-Ross' framework has been taught now to generations of medical students and other helping professionals, resulting in it becoming a cornerstone of our thinking about grief as a process.

Presenting grief in this way, as a series of normal and expectable stages to be negotiated, offered the gift of acknowledging the deeply human process of adjustment to a reality that is life changing, whether that centered on the imminence of one's own death or the mourning of the loss of another. The downside of stage models like Kubler-Ross', however, is that may be seen as prescriptive of the feelings and process of grief, telling people in mourning or those observing or helping them, in effect, what is "normal." Such structured theories run the risk of being reified and interfering with the actual lived experience of the bereaved. For example, misusing Kubler-Ross' stages, grieving people have been told things like "You can't have accepted the reality of the loss yet. You haven't bargained or gotten depressed."

In a related vein, Worden (1991) proposed that there are four tasks of mourning that must be completed for the process to be resolved. Worden suggests that the bereaved must first accept the reality of the loss. This is followed by the need to work through the pain of grief. Third, the bereaved must adjust to the absence of the deceased in the environment. Finally, the person in mourning must move on with a new life while finding a lasting connection to the deceased.

In response to the possible rigidity of stage models, two other frameworks have been proposed that conceptualize grief as more fluid and individualized. The first of these, known as the dual process model (Stroebe & Schut, 2010), considers the relationship of the bereaved to two perspectives with respect to the loss. These are referred to as loss orientation and restoration orientation. As the name suggests, Stroebe and Schut (2010) view grieving individuals as engaged in both of these processes in an overlapping and perhaps alternating way. At times the bereaved may find themselves preoccupied by the pain of their loss and their effort to manage the absence of the beloved (loss orientation); at other times they may find that their energy is more focused on staying active and reengaging in the world, investing in the discovery of what their life moving forward will look like (restoration orientation). The particular balance and flow of loss orientation and restoration orientation will be unique to the individual.

In contrast to the ambivalence inherent in the dual process model in which the bereaved move back and forth between the two orientations to loss, Rubin's (1999) two track model offers a perspective on grief as unfolding on parallel, simultaneous tracks. The first, the biopsychosocial track, is centered on the physical and emotional manifestations of grief and loss as well as the repercussions the bereaved experience in the social world as they renegotiate their connections to others. The second, the relational track, pertains to the internal reworking of the relationship to the one who was lost. This unfolds as memories and stories are revisited, the loss is memorialized in some ways, and the nature of one's sense of ongoing connectedness to the deceased is established at least in a preliminary way.

Take a moment to think about the way that each of these theoretical approaches tells a story of sorts about what is happening within and around us as we process the experience of grief. Let's consider one more point of view. The model that perhaps most fully reflects our narrative perspective, rooted in social constructionism as we have discussed it, is expressed in the extensive work of Robert Neimeyer and his colleagues (Neimeyer, 2001a, 2001b, 2005, 2006). Neimeyer's scholarship and practice are centered on the reconstruction of meaning in the wake of loss, the effort to integrate the experience of the loss into what I have referred to as the story of our selves, the world, and our selves in the world. Narrative is ideally suited to this effort to make meaning of the often life-changing nature of loss inasmuch as it "specializes in the forging of links between the exceptional and the ordinary" (Bruner, 1990, p. 47). We will review this body of work in some detail throughout the chapter.

Meaning Reconstruction in Narratives of Grief and Loss

Narrative is, if you will, the armature or skeleton that gives shape to the meaning we make of experience. The stories we tell ourselves provide the vehicle that allows us to structure the sequence of our life's events and to put them in a broader context that frames their significance. As we have discussed, this storytelling emerges from within us, from our own meaning making instinct. But it is also shaped by the social context in which we are immersed. In addition to being an important medium through which we relate to that world, it is the way we relate to ourselves. It undergirds the countless interpretations of experience that are interwoven to inform our identity.

Natalya was a 23-year-old young woman who came for treatment for the severe anxiety that had limited her functioning for years. She had been home schooled for the second and third years of high school because of the intensity of her anxiety when she tried to leave the house. With in-home therapy and medication Natalya had made enough progress that she was able to attend school for her senior year. When I met her she was a second-year university student studying biology, and the anxiety was returning, sometimes rendering her unable to get out of her car to go to class. This was what Natalya and I worked on principally in her therapy, so I was curious when a different issue moved to the forefront of our sessions.

I knew from my initial assessment that Natalya had been born in the former Soviet Union. Her father was a military officer who died in his early 40s when she was just 5 years old. She told me that he had been an alcoholic and that his early death was caused by medical complications that resulted from his drinking. She had not been aware of this as a small child, but her mother had told her stories of his life and of his death. Following the collapse of the Soviet Union, Natalya's mother had the opportunity to come to the United States and emigrated with her sister and young Natalya. The three women lived in a small apartment together until Natalya's aunt eventually married and moved out on her own. Now it was just Natalya and her mother. Though her mother spoke some English, they spoke Russian at home. For Natalya, having immigrated so young, English was now the dominant language in which she lived and thought.

During one session Natalya began to talk about memories of her father. They were simply memories of everyday life, at least as she recalled them in our session. Natalya became quite reflective and began to talk about what it felt like to grow up without her father. She thought of the special occasions when she was particularly aware of his absence, and of missing his presence in the ordinariness of life. What would it have been like just to have him around, to be part of her growing up, to get to know him as an adult, and to have him know her? Natalya paused and said in an off-handed way, "It's sort of ironic for me to sit here and think about these things. I've never even been a good daughter to him." It was clear to me that there was something important underlying Natalya's statement about herself.

"What do you mean when you say you weren't a good daughter to your father?"
She paused.
"I've never said this out loud … but I don't think I really loved my father. So what kind of daughter am I?"
"You believe that you didn't love your father?"
"Yeah. Not really. I think of him and if I'm being honest, I feel nothing. I tell people about him; I've even talked about his death with friends, boyfriends, you know … And nothing. I don't feel anything."
"So what does that mean to you?"
"Well, think about it? What kind of daughter doesn't feel anything for her father? I think about him dying; I remember the day he died. I think about his funeral and the day we left Russia to come to the United States. I remember thinking, 'I'm leaving him here. I'm leaving my father behind.' My mother said, 'Your father will always be with us. No matter where we are.' But I don't feel anything."
We sat together in silence for a few moments. She continued.
"Do you know I don't even cry for him? Never. When I think of him or talk about him … A good daughter would cry."
Note how Natalya is aware of socially constructed narratives of what it means to be a "good daughter" who loves her father, and the story she tells about herself and her relationship to him based on the meaning she makes of her absence of feeling.
I asked her, "How long have you felt this way, Natalya? How long have you carried around this sense of being a bad daughter?"
"As long as I can remember I guess. Since I was a little girl."
"You were five years old when you came to the United States. Is that right?"
"Yeah. I was five."
"Did you speak English when you came to here?"
"No. Only Russian. In fact it was hard in kindergarten because I didn't speak English at all at first and it wasn't like there were a whole lot of Russian speakers roaming around my school. But I learned it quickly."
Though I wasn't certain about it, I had an idea.
I asked Natalya, "Would you try an experiment with me?"
She seemed cautious but curious and with a slight grin said ok.
"I would like you to tell me about the death of your father. But I want you to tell me in Russian."
Natalya laughed. "But you don't speak Russian!"
"Correct. Not a word," I said. "Just indulge me."

Natalya paused, thinking of where to begin. Then she spoke—beautiful, fluent Russian. And I listened. At first she looked at me, speaking directly to me. Eventually though, her attention was drawn inward, as though she were telling the story of her father's death to an inner audience—to herself. Though I couldn't understand a word, I could see and hear her storytelling becoming more animated, more intense.

Within a few moments, I could see Natalya's eyes begin to moisten. When the first tear rolled down her cheek, she looked at me, her story uninterrupted. Her tears began to flow more freely, and more quickly. The words caught in her throat and, as she continued, she began to sob heavily. After a time there were no more words, only tears.

A few minutes later, when she had regained her composure, Natalya looked at me, stunned and confused.

"What just happened?" she asked. "Where did that all come from?"

"From you." I answered. "That's your story."

I continued. "When you were just a little girl who was going through the death of her father, you didn't speak English, only Russian. So the way you initially told that story to yourself and tried to make sense of it and of all your feelings was in Russian. That's the way it was actually encoded in your brain. When you came to the United States you learned English, but it's hard to relate to that memory in another language. We can speak the words and recount events, but it doesn't link up with the part of our brain, the part of ourselves where our emotional experience lies. You can tell the story, but it's like having a filter on. You just don't feel it in the same way."[1]

Natalya sat, trying to absorb what I was saying. I returned to her narrative of her father and her self.

"All these years, you have told yourself the story that you were a bad daughter who didn't love her father because there was no sadness and no tears. But you were just telling the story – his story, your story – in the wrong language."

In whatever language we think, and speak, and feel, the stories we tell about grief and loss, as well as any other human experience for that matter, are infused with the meaning we make of those events. And our meaning making, in turn, contributes to the form and focus of our story. These are not just the stories of the loss itself, but of what it says about us, our identity, and our life as we understand it.

In her book *The Year of Magical Thinking*, Joan Didion (2006b) writes with pained eloquence of the sudden death of her husband of 40 years, John Gregory Dunne. On December 30, 2003, Dunne sustained a massive heart attack in the couple's New York apartment as they prepared to sit down to dinner. Didion writes,

Grief turns out to be a place none of us know until we reach it. We anticipate (we know) that someone close to us could die, but we do not look beyond the few days or weeks that immediately follow such an imagined death. We misconstrue the nature of even those few days or weeks ... We have no way of knowing that the funeral itself will be anodyne, a kind of narcotic regression in which we are wrapped in the care of others and the gravity and meaning of the occasion. Nor can we know ahead of the fact (and here lies the heart of the difference between grief as we imagine it and grief as it is) the unending absence that follows, the void, the very opposite of meaning, the relentless succession of moments during which we will confront the experience of meaninglessness itself. (pp. 188–189)

This is, of course, the narrative challenge of grief and loss—to find ourselves in that void, in the meaninglessness that renders life so disorienting, and makes us feel that we have lost even our very selves and the orientation of our life. If you've ever had occasion to swim or even just wade in the ocean, you've likely had the experience of a wave suddenly inundating you, crashing over your head, knocking you off your feet, and turning you, for what might be a frightening few moments, completely upside down. We generally do regain our footing, and as we surface from that turbulent water we catch our breath and reorient ourselves to the world around us.

---

[1] For more on this understanding of the role of language for the bilingual client, cf. Foster (1998).

Grief is something like that. As we make our way through the upheaval it causes in our life, our storytelling is there to help us find our way again. Narrative is the profoundly and uniquely human tool we use, not to get back to where we were—that is not possible—but to find our way forward. Neimeyer (2016a) discusses the nature of the grieving process as an "attempt to reaffirm or reconstruct a world of meaning that has been challenged by loss" (p. 212). This is part and parcel of the renegotiation of the narrative of the self. Neimeyer (2004) has referred to this as the effort to integrate a micro-narrative from everyday life into the macro-narrative of our life as a whole. In other words, we take the story of our particular loss and fit it into the overarching story we tell about our life, the world, and ourselves.

You may remember from Chap. 3 on trauma narrative that Park and Folkman (1997) conceptualized this as the relationship between situational meaning and global meaning. The interaction between these dimensions of meaning making is a process of assimilation and accommodation. Assimilation refers to the ability to *fit* an experience, in this case a loss over which we are grieving, into the overall meaning making framework that governs our life. When, however, the loss is too great or challenges us too deeply to simply fit into our schema of life and the world, then we must *accommodate* it by altering our global sense of meaning.

You may also recognize similarities in this thinking to the work of Janoff-Bulman (Janoff-Bulman, 1992, 2006; Janoff-Bulman & Frantz, 1997) that we also discussed in Chap. 3. Recall that Janoff-Bulman writes of the way trauma, and in the present context loss, may shatter the basic assumptions we have about the world. She suggests that we intuitively engage in a process of renegotiation whereby we may reestablish a sense of meaning and order in life. Put in other terms, we work to reestablish the coherence of the narrative we tell about life and the world in order to go on living. Returning to the work of Joan Didion for a moment, in what may seem like an apt coincidence, you might find it interesting to know that a volume of her collected nonfiction was named for the first line of her essay "The White Album." The book is entitled *We Tell Ourselves Stories in Order to Live* (Didion, 2006a).

Didion is, of course, not the only author to attempt to portray the experience of grief in words. In fact, many have done so, sometimes in ways that have given us an enduring testimony to the power of loss. C.S. Lewis (1961) penned the now classic, *A Grief Observed*, a recounting of his experience of grief following the death of his wife Joy, referred to in the book as *H* for her true first name, Helen. Lewis writes,

> I think I am beginning to understand why grief feels like suspense. It comes from the frustration of so many impulses that had become habitual. Thought after thought, feeling after feeling, action after action, had H. for their object. Now their target is gone. I keep on through habit fitting an arrow to the string, then I remember and have to lay the bow down. So many roads lead thought to H. I set out on one of them. But now there's an impassable frontierpost across it. So many roads once; now so many *culs de sac*. (p. 47)

One of the gifts of such descriptions of the lived reality of grief is that it reminds those living with the pain of loss that, in spite of the suffering it causes, there is something normal and expectable about that pain. What's more, the vast majority of people do move at their own pace on a course toward healing that will bring with it a newly integrated story about life and loss. What, then, of the times when this kind of healing journey does not seem to be moving forward? How do we differentiate between what we refer to as *normal grief* and *complicated grief*? It is to this distinction that we now turn.

Differentiating Normal Grief and Complicated Grief

One of the ideas we have been considering in this chapter is that each of us has a story about the meaning and nature of grief and loss. It may be based on extensive experience of grief or, frankly, little to no experience. It might stem from stories we have heard of others who have suffered the pain of loss, or even media portrayals of the bereaved and what it means to lose someone. However we came by it, we each have a story, and part of the fabric of that story is some sense of what grief looks and feels like, as well as how it unfolds. In other words, we tell ourselves and each other a story about what is "normal." By inevitable contrast, then, we also have a story about what does not seem "normal." Because we are social constructionists, this formulation is riddled with problems. What does it mean to be normal, feel normal, grieve normally, or react normally to loss? Nonetheless, with those questions to keep us humble, we can begin to look at that part of our collective social narrative that does have something to say about the expectable course and variations of grief, as well as the ways in which certain patterns of grief become concerning. After all, for all of the ways our individuality results in narratives that are personal and unique, we also have a great deal in common. The ability to honor the individuality of the person in front of us as well as to appreciate the ways in which we are alike in our human living is the very thing that helps us connect and reminds us that we are not alone.

An early effort to describe the symptomatology of grief from a clinical point of view came from Lindemann (1944) whose study of 101 bereaved patients (including survivors of the famous Cocoanut Grove fire and many family members of the deceased) led to his portrayal of acute grief as featuring somatic complaints, a preoccupation with the image of the person who died, guilt, hostility, and a noticeable change of routine. Thankfully, the majority of those who suffer this acute form of grief notice that their symptoms gradually resolve, and that while there may always be a certain sensitivity to their experience of loss, they are able to return to an adequate level of functioning that is not affected by debilitating grief. This resilience in the face of grief is remarkably common, with 85–90% of the bereaved relying on their own instincts as well as the coping mechanisms and supports available to them to find their way through (Bonanno, 2009; Bonanno, Westphal, & Mancini, 2011).

Yet we know that for some bereaved individuals, the experience of grief is more intractable. Earlier in this chapter we considered one view of this that I referred to as complicated grief, defined as "grieving that fails to move forward adaptively as the person integrates the loss, instead remaining intense, preoccupying, prolonged, and life-limiting" (Neimeyer & Harris, 2016, p. 163). Elsewhere, this has been characterized as prolonged grief disorder (PGD) (Peri, Hasson-Ohayon, Garber, Tuval-Mashiach, & Boelen, 2016), a category proposed for inclusion in the eleventh revision of the International Classification of Diseases (ICD-11) (Maercker et al., 2013). PGD is conceptualized as a grief that is debilitating in an ongoing way and may include "painful yearning for the deceased, separation anxiety, difficulties accepting the loss, and difficulties engaging in new activities after the loss" (Maercker & Lalor, 2012 as cited in Peri et al. 2016, p. 1). In general, we may begin to think of these intense kinds of grief reactions as problematic for the bereaved if they extend beyond the 6-month mark post-loss. This is not intended to pathologize the grieving, but to call attention to the kinds of support individuals may need if their difficulty coping with emotions and functioning in daily life continues for this long. Once again, this is likely to be true in only 10–15% of cases (Neimeyer & Harris, 2016; Peri et al., 2016).

Let's take a moment at this point, to reflect explicitly on a dimension of grief and loss that we have been alluding to, but have not explored fully. We have discussed how, from a social constructionist point of view, narratives emerge not only from the internal story-making process of the individual, but also from the social environment in which they are embedded. Recall Bruner's (1986, 1987, 1990) notion that culture, the social context, sets the range of possible interpretations of experience that shape the formation of our narratives. It is these shared meanings that inform our storytelling. Here we are referring to culture on the broadest level as well as the numerous subcultures to which we belong by virtue of the various identifications we espouse.

In the context of grief and loss, the meanings we make of bereavement are informed by this social context. As Neimeyer (2005) notes, we all seek the validation of our interpretation of experience in culturally endorsed ways. This means that we signal to each other within our cultures and subcultures what the meaning of loss is, how it is to be processed appropriately, and what a healthy response to it looks and feels like (Neimeyer, Klass, & Dennis, 2014). This notion informs the way in which we mourn. What is the right balance between public and private mourning? With whom do we share our pain, how often, and for how long? What aspects of it are appropriate to share and which are best kept private? Our responses to all of these questions are shaped by the multiple layers of context and culture (including race, ethnicity, age, class, gender, etc.) that make up the particular world in which we live and experience the pain of our grief. In return, these responses shape our interpretation of our selves and the meaning we make of our experience, as well as the others' narratives about our bereavement.

To the extent that our bereavement conforms to the expectable course prescribed by my culture(s), I am likely to feel validated and supported. However, the opposite is perhaps also true. To the extent my personal process of grief does not follow that socially endorsed path, I may feel isolated, confused, and even more at odds with myself and others. It is important to note, of course, that support and validation are not binary (e.g., yes/no) variables. They are not either present or absent. Rather, they exist on a continuum. We may feel *more* or *less* supported and validated. This degree of support, we may find, is related to the degree to which I grieve in those socially endorsed ways. In my clinical experience, there are nearly endless permutations to this general principle based on the unique situation of every client. Some may recount how there are certain people in their life (a spouse, a friend, a sibling) who they feel are truly there for them, no matter what. Others have been overcome by the outpouring of support from those from whom they would have least expected it. Still others, and a fair number of them in my experience, will tell you that those closest to them have struggled to remain supportive and to understand what they are going through and how.

In Chap. 3 I told you the story of Catherine, my client whose son had committed suicide and who wore a charm with his image around her neck. Catherine suffered from a prolonged, complicated grief, one that felt to her like it had dug in and planted roots. It held on to her and, in some ways, she held on to it. She didn't know how else to do it. One of the complicating factors for Catherine was that her family had communicated to her verbally and nonverbally that they didn't want to hear it anymore. They had to move on. Of course, they were grieving as well. Catherine's protracted, unresolved mourning was a constant painful reminder to them of the unspeakable loss they had all experienced. Her ongoing pain made them feel too raw. They weren't cold or insensitive; they just couldn't tolerate the grief any more.

I suggest that it is important to try to maintain this kind of balance when thinking about clients and their families and other social supports. There is no doubt that our clients are sometimes surrounded by bad people and bad situations. There is no doubt that many of our clients just have not received what they need from the environment in order to grow and thrive. More often than not, however, I find that people are trying their best. In Catherine's case, for example, her family and friends were good people simply brought to the limits of their own abilities to support Catherine and to cope themselves.

This brings us to an important point not only with respect to Catherine, but also perhaps large portions of contemporary Western culture. That is, we have great difficulty dealing with sadness and emotional pain. I am not taking the position of an anthropologist here, much less a historian. My point is not to compare and contrast how different cultures cope with such pain either presently or in the past. Rather, it is to note as a clinician and social scientist the extraordinary lengths to which our culture will go to avoid the ultimately inescapable reality of pain and loss. We are uncomfortable with our own pain and that of others. On systemic levels, it has been suggested that we have pathologized ordinary sadness (Horowitz & Wakefield, 2007), and that the pharmaceutical industry has profited mightily from our difficulty living with our emotional discomfort. It is clearly true that there are large numbers of people who have benefitted from advances in pharmacology that have diminished or eliminated symptoms of depression and anxiety that had previously been crippling. This, in my view, is beyond question. Medicine can often be an invaluable tool for our clients' well-being. In a broader cultural sense, however, we seek escape from sadness and other forms of emotional discomfort in any number of distractions including work, drugs, alcohol, sex, as well as internal defenses such as repression, denial, projection, and a host of others. We pursue our own image of youth and beauty at enormous cost, both literally and metaphorically. Advances in science and technology seduce us into fantasizing that we can stave off what we (including physicians, nurses, therapists, and scientists) have always known, and that in the end grief and loss touch us all.

It is into this mix, then, of the public and the private, the widely shared and the highly idiosyncratic, that we step as social workers with our grieving clients. It is a sacred ground, I think, where we meet them at perhaps their most vulnerable, taking seriously the trust they place in us when they invite us into such a delicate part of their life as the losses they mourn. As we wait with patient attention for them to recount their story, we contribute important parts of the context for our work. We communicate perhaps with words, but even with our presence that we are prepared to receive their story. That we can take it. That we will honor their story, even the pieces that confuse and maybe frighten them, that they can't present to us all worked out, polished up, and tied with a perfect bow. We assure them that we will listen deeply, and search with them for understanding and the meaning of their story in all its complexity.

This often entails creating with our clients a space where they can work through especially difficult questions and feelings. They may be feeling ambivalent about the loss they are mourning (Alves et al., 2016). In my experience clients often feel some degree of pressure, generated either from within based on their personal history or from those around them, to feel *one* way, respond *one* way to the loss. There is some intuitive appeal to the simplicity of having one emotional response to a loss. It is neater and seems more manageable. But I have rarely known this to be the case. More often, we human beings are a bundle of multiple emotions and meanings at once (Worden, 1991). In addition to the sadness of missing someone they love who has died, clients may feel angry with them. They may question whether there is more they could or should have done for that person. They may feel desperate to heal, but also guilty, wondering if doing so would somehow call into question their love and the genuineness of their mourning. Similarly, they may feel a deep sense of relief at the end of a long, painful process of dying, but judge themselves unfaithful then to their lost loved one.

I recall a woman who spent almost all day, every day for weeks caring for her dying mother. There were countless hours of sitting by her bedside, at first talking with her and tending to her needs, then after she had slipped into unconsciousness, waiting, the sound of an unwatched television show droning in the background, the fluorescent lights of the room straining her eyes and making her feel even more tired than she knew she already was. The waiting was exhausting. I saw her just a few days after her mother died. The funeral was finally over. She told me about it all. She told me how everyone present expressed their admiration for what a wonderful daughter she was, how faithful she had been to her mother right until the very end. "But do you want to know something?" she said. "Do you want to know what I was really thinking in the moments after my mother died? That all I wanted was to go home, take a long hot shower, and clean my house. I hadn't done a thing for weeks except sit with my mother. All I wanted now was to clean my house and to put some order back in my life."

She was mourning her mother to be sure, but she was also craving a clean house, a metaphor for the restoration of order, control, and predictability that had been so absent from that vigil by her mother's bedside. Though her reaction was entirely understandable she struggled with this mix of emotions and what people would think of her if they knew. Loss is like this. It evokes a host of different responses based on the nature of the loss, the history of those involved, the circumstances under which it happens, and the meanings it calls into question (Volkan & Zintl, 1993). It may involve actual death, or another type of loss entirely. Let's turn our attention now to the varieties of loss that we may encounter in our practice and of which we need to be aware.

The Varieties of Loss

One of the points we have been discussing is the virtually innumerable ways in which loss may present itself in our life, setting off a process of grieving that we must negotiate. Any effort to elaborate a comprehensive list of the varieties of loss that a social worker may face would be futile. Having said that, I would like to offer a brief overview of some of the losses that I believe are important for us to be attentive to as social workers. This kind of attention is especially important since clients will not always make a connection on their own between a particular kind of distress they are feeling (especially if it comes some time later) and a loss they have sustained. Our ability to hear that theme in their narrative and potentially to help them make that connection may be of great significance.

The loss of a child is one that is widely acknowledged to be potentially devastating to parents, siblings, and extended family and community. It is important to be mindful of the number of forms this kind of loss can take. We may grieve the death of a child following a prolonged illness such as cancer (Price & Jones, 2015). The way in which the course of the illness unfolds can contribute greatly to the challenge of making meaning for the bereaved. Similarly, gender differences may be noted in the way fathers and mothers process the loss (McGoldrick, 2004). This can create the possibility of added friction in the relationship between parents as well as between parents and the siblings of the deceased if variations on mourning are not recognized and understood. The intensity of the pain of such a loss may result in survivors feeling isolated when those around them simply don't know what to say or how to be present. From a treatment point of view, sustained support in anticipation of the loss may be helpful to the family in managing the protracted nature of the experience (Price & Jones, 2015; Tan, Docherty, Barfield, & Brandon, 2012).

The experience of losing a child suddenly due to an accident or some other lethal event may overwhelm families in a different way inasmuch as they are given no preparation for the loss (Lichtenthal, Neimeyer, Currier, Roberts, & Jordan, 2013). Loved ones are thrust into a confusing vortex of emotions and details, having to respond to numerous aspects of the reality of the loss and decisions that need to be made all at once. Such a rupture to the anticipated orderliness of our life narrative can be arresting (Crossley, 2000, 2003).

Many years ago while working in a hospital, I entered a room on the children's ward to find a small boy, Tyler, lying in the bed seemingly asleep. His mother, Melissa, was sitting in a chair staring out the window. She turned when I came in. I introduced myself and told her I was there to be helpful in any way I could. She joined me at Tyler's bedside, told me his name, and took his hand. Tyler was 4 years old. Just over a week earlier, he was playing in the backyard of their home. It was summer time, and Tyler had a lot of toys outside including a swing set and jungle gym. He loved being outside. Melissa was in the kitchen cleaning up from dinner. At some point she realized that she didn't hear Tyler playing. She looked out the window but didn't see him immediately. Calling his name, she stepped out into the yard. That was when she saw him. She screamed his name, screamed for her husband Mike, and started running.

Several days before, they had had a tree service come to take down a large tree in the yard. The workers had cut the tree into large cylindrical pieces and left them on their sides until they could be carted away. As best as Melissa could tell, Tyler must have been playing with one of those pieces when it began to roll. It was now lying directly on Tyler's small chest. His eyes were closed. He was not struggling or making a sound. He did not appear to be breathing. Mike had now arrived and immediately rolled the tree section off his son. Melissa went to call 911. Tyler was in fact not breathing, and Mike began doing CPR until the EMTs arrived. Within moments they were on their way to the hospital; one EMT continued compressions and breaths.

By the time the ambulance got to the hospital, Melissa and Mike following right behind, Tyler's heart was beating and he was breathing. They cried with relief. Later that day, however, after extensive testing, they received crushing news. It seemed that Tyler was wedged under that log, deprived of oxygen, long enough that he suffered catastrophic brain damage. In fact, the only portion of Tyler's brain that continued to function was his brain stem, responsible for the maintenance of his vital processes such as respiration and heart rate. The doctor assured them that Tyler was in no pain, but that it was not possible for him to emerge from his current state of unconsciousness.

Melissa and Mike were beside themselves with grief. It was as if a tornado had swept in and overturned their world in an instant. Over the course of the first few days there were oceans of tears, rage against the tree service for leaving the tree in such large pieces especially with a small child around, a simultaneous clinging to family and friends, and wishing that everyone would go away. There was hope that the doctors were wrong—maybe there would be a miracle—as well as the nauseating feeling that they were right. And there was blame, and finger pointing. "Why weren't you watching him?" "Well, what were *you* doing?"

As Melissa and I talked, Mike arrived from work. He had taken off from work the first few days, and he and Melissa had stayed in the hospital around the clock, watching and waiting. But eventually he had to go back to work. He was out of sick and vacation time, and they really needed the money. He came to the hospital every day after work, tried to give Melissa a break, and sat in silence with Tyler.

I got to know Melissa and Mike better over the next couple of weeks. There was palpable tension between them. In one of our early conversations they shared with me that they had been on the verge of separating even before the accident. Mike had been sleeping on the couch for weeks. This all just made things worse. As if this weren't enough, they also found themselves in two different places with respect to Tyler and his condition. They were telling themselves two very different narratives. This came to a head when the medical team met with them to offer their recommendation that Tyler's nutrition and hydration be discontinued. Because Tyler's brain stem was working normally, it was possible that he could live for years in his persistent vegetative state.

Tyler as they knew him was gone, but his body could continue to function indefinitely if he was given water and nutrients. There would be no suffering, and no pain for Tyler. The effects, the doctor assured them, would not even be noticeable from the outside. Melissa and Mike both rejected the idea as horrible and unimaginable, but after a few days, the differences in the stories they were telling themselves began to emerge and the conflict and bitterness between them grew. Mike was in favor of withdrawing nutrition and hydration, but Melissa refused. He threatened to take her to court, while she would file a countersuit.

When I was able to get them in a room together, I tried to draw out from each of them the story they were telling themselves about what lay ahead and the implications of those stories for the different choices they could make. Melissa's story was of the faithful mother who would not give up on her child when everyone else was ready to. But it was more than that. It was the story of a mother who, if she went along with the doctor's recommendations, might be filled with regret, always wondering what might have been if she had waited just 1 more day, 1 more week. It was the story of a mother who would never know if a miracle might have been given to them. For his part, Mike told the story of a father who was devastated, who didn't know how to go on. It was the story of a father who lived with a pit in his stomach and who went to work every day not knowing if his son would be alive or dead when he got home. Mike paused and corrected himself. He felt in his bones that Tyler was already gone. He was just waiting for Tyler's body to give out. Melissa couldn't let go; Mike needed this part of the story to end.

There was no way out of the situation that was causing them such pain. There were only ways through. Listening to each other's story softened some of the immediate tension between them. They were both suffering; they both loved their son. They were both trying to figure out what was best for him. In the end, they did decide to remove nutrition and hydration from Tyler. They took him home where nurses and aids helped them throughout the day and night. Less than a week later, I got a call from Melissa and Mike saying that Tyler had passed. They knew they had a long road of grief ahead of them and that there were supports and resources available to them, which they planned on making use of.

Still another type of loss of a child comes in the case of miscarriage, stillbirth, and fetal loss (Fernadez, Harris, & Leschied, 2011; Jones, 2015; McCreight, 2008; Neimeyer, 2016b; Sawicka, 2016). Like the death of a child due to illness or accident, these losses involve the added mourning for an imagined future that will not come to pass both for the child and for the parents. Unfortunately, families that sustain this kind of loss often find that there is insufficient awareness and support for their experience of grief (Sawicka, 2016) and that their pain is underestimated or unrecognized (Boss, 2010). This may be particularly true for fathers who have lost children in this way (McCreight, 2004).

Clearly, a number of other losses may be significant to all the members of a family. Not only does this imply that each member may have his or her own specific reaction to the loss based on their relationship to the deceased and their place in the structure of the family, but the dynamics within the family as a whole and their collective narrative as a family may be altered as well (Baddeley & Singer, 2010). Loss of a sibling may be life changing, not just in one's childhood or youth, but even later in life as the sibling relationship may come to stand out from others in unique ways (Sveen, Eilegard, Steineck, & Kreicbergs, 2014; Wright, 2016). Loss of a parent is a meaningful event at any point in the life span, whether the survivor is of advanced age himself or herself, in their youth and adolescence, or anywhere in between (Stikkelbroek, Bodden, Reitz, Vollerbergh, & van Baar, 2016). Loss of a spouse may be similarly significant, with the unique meaning of the loss shaped by the context of the particular marital relationship and the timing of the death (Walsh & McGoldrick, 2004).

Outside the context of the biological family, there are any number of relationships in which a death can lead to significant mourning and a change to our narrative and way of making meaning. This can occur in the context of an important friendship, a relationship to a teacher or mentor, or even one's therapist (Cornell, 2014). On a larger social level, we may find ourselves mourning a loss collectively as was the case following the assassination of John F. Kennedy or the attacks on the United States on September 11, 2001 (Kitch, 2003).

The circumstances of a death also contribute to its meaning both personally and in the social world. Loss as a result of violence may be particularly hard to metabolize and may present an additional challenge to our efforts to reestablish meaning through the use of narrative (Currier & Neimeyer, 2007). As we have seen so frequently in the media, violent deaths may spark the outrage not only of family members but also of the broader community (Aldrich & Kallivayalil, 2016). However, the community's attention to the needs of those most personally bereaved may fade well before those needs are fulfilled, and those most deeply affected may feel forgotten after public interest has waned. A similar dynamic may be seen following a loss to suicide when survivors struggle to understand the decision of a loved one who took their own life and to find meaning in a context that often feels very isolating (Pritchard & Buckle, 2017; Sands, Jordan, & Neimeyer, 2010). As we discussed in Chap. 3, organizations such as the American Foundation for Suicide Prevention (www.afsp.org) work not only to raise awareness and prevent suicide, but also to support survivors dealing with a loss that so often remains in the shadows.

There are other experiences of loss that are often relegated to the margins, resulting in what we refer to as disenfranchised grief, stigmatized loss, or ambiguous loss (Boss, 2010; Doka, 2002; Werner-Lin & Moro, 2004). We saw that this is sometimes true in the case of miscarriages, stillbirths, and fetal loss. It has also been true over time of same-sex couples when one partner was inhibited from expressing their grief or received no support upon the death of their partner either because the relationship had not been publicly acknowledged or because their rights as partner or spouse were not legally recognized. Men and women who had spent decades with their significant other were turned away, for example, in hospitals—told that medical information could only be given to a member of the family.

In a similar way, families of men and women who died of AIDS have had their grief silenced because of stigma (Werner-Lin & Moro, 2004). I once went to be with the family of a man with AIDS when they gathered at the hospital on the morning of his death. As I entered the room and greeted the family, the man's two brothers came toward me quickly and asked me to step outside with them. In the hallway they thanked me for coming but wanted me to know that they were the only ones who were aware that their brother had AIDS. Everyone else in the room, including the deceased man's parents, thought he had cancer. They said that this was the way their brother wanted it. They had lived with the secret ever since he was diagnosed several years earlier. I reassured them that I would certainly respect their wishes, and also told them that if they would like to talk privately at some point about their own experience of loss I would be more than happy to do so. The family was grieving, and they were supporting each other in their mourning. But these two men had accompanied their brother from the moment he was found to be HIV+, through his experience of AIDS, and ultimately to his death. They had each other to rely on, and they did, but there was nowhere they felt free to talk about their story and the way they made meaning both of their brother's death and the silence and stigma that surrounded it.

Finally, the narrative implications of end-of-life and palliative care are extensive enough to warrant an in-depth treatment that is beyond the scope of this chapter. For our present purposes I'd like simply to offer a couple of points for your consideration. First, the end of life, to the extent that it is anticipated, is a key time of renegotiation of the story of one's life and the meaning of one's journey. For seniors, this commonly and importantly takes the form of life review, a revisiting and retelling of one's story with a view to coalescing its meaning as a whole (Butler, 1963; Westerhof & Bohlmeijer, 2014). Life review is a moment of integration that calls upon us to listen attentively and to bear witness to this exercise in meaning making.

Second, in addition to being a time when the story of how one has lived is reviewed, end-of-life reflection commonly includes a formulation of how one would like to die and the meaning of that as well. At times, these choices can create conflict in families either because one or more members disagree with the wishes of the dying member or because family members find themselves at odds with each other over "what is best" for their loved one. The increasing commonality, and in some instances the requirement, of advance directives such as a power of attorney or living will may be seen as an effort to avoid this kind of conflict, and to ensure that a person's final days will conform as closely as possible to the narrative of their wishes (Gillespie, 2017; Tadel, 2014).

Losses Not Involving Physical Death

We have explored so far in this chapter the varieties of grief and loss that we may encounter around the experience of death. However, actual physical death is not the only kind of loss, even if it is one that will touch us all at some point. There are, in fact, many other ways in which we encounter loss in life and are brought to an experience of mourning and the need to make meaning through the stories we tell ourselves and each other. Given what we know about the personal and social elements that contribute to our experience of loss, let's consider some of the many losses we will encounter in practice that do not involve physical death.

Reminders of our own mortality and the limitations of our human bodies are put before us all the time. And while such experiences (e.g., feeling the general effects of aging) remind us that none of us is given forever in this world, some occurrences drive that awareness home more powerfully. Consider, for example, the experience of paralysis following spinal cord injury and the impact of this not only on one's physical capabilities but also on one's sense of self, and the multiple roles one plays in life from worker to parent to spouse (Clifton, 2014). Also of a physical nature we may think of the impact of hysterectomy or mastectomy on the narratives of self of the women who require them (Collis, 2007; Piot-Ziegler, Sassi, Raffoul, & Delaloye, 2010). This kind of loss involves the body and its appearance, but it may also touch upon their sense of the social constructs of womanhood and femininity and the way they are seen in the world. Additionally, depending on the timing and circumstances, hysterectomy will impact the dimension of a women's self-narrative as childbearing. Issues of infertility similarly evoke feelings of grief for both men and women. Each of these experiences may involve a highly personalized mourning on both social (including relationships with romantic partners or spouses) and individual levels.

In a different way, living with a brain injury can impact not only the story of the individual (if their story-making ability is not interfered with) but those around them who may feel that their loved one has been more or less profoundly changed by their injury. Similar dynamics are encountered around a diagnosis of dementia—whether one's own or that of a loved one. The anticipation of one's very sense of identity growing dimmer or the witnessing of a beloved parent, spouse, or sibling becoming increasingly unrecognizable in their personality is a particularly painful form of loss. This is a change to the story both of what has been as memories of a shared narrative fade and of what was hoped for, as the promise of the future grows less promising (Boss, 1999, 2010).

As social workers, we frequently are called upon to sit with clients' sense of grief over life events and circumstances that are unrelated to their physical health. One may think, for example, of divorce or the end of a relationship, and the loss of a future that one anticipated for oneself. This can be true for either partner, but may take on a particular meaning when the end of the relationship is not one's choice. Indeed, the loss of a dream and the vision of the life one wanted to live can cause profound feelings of mourning and can challenge the coherence of one's narrative of self, significant others, and the world. Other examples of this include the renegotiation that may occur at midlife and similar experiences that represent challenges to one's narcissism (Goldstein, 2005). Job loss and a change of financial status and outlook can also be serious narcissistic losses that may result in upheaval in one's story which can occur at any age.

A young Caucasian man in his mid-20s named Joe came for treatment at an urban mental health clinic where I was working. He told me right at the outset that he would have much preferred to see a therapist in private practice where he believed he would have gotten a superior kind of treatment. This wasn't possible, however, because he had Medicaid. Joe was unable to find a practitioner near his suburban town who would take Medicaid and he could not afford to pay for treatment out of pocket. He complained of significant symptoms of depression and anxiety that had been haunting him for years. He did not work because of his condition. He tried taking college classes but had gotten no momentum, due in part to his emotional state and in part to the need to take out student loans and accrue debt.

When I asked him to tell me about the story of his depression and anxiety, Joe took me back to his senior year of high school. At the time he lived in one of the wealthier sections of an upscale town. His family had a sizeable piece property; in addition to the "main house," they also had a carriage house at the gate that was used as guest quarters and occasionally as a home office space for his father. Joe's father worked in the banking industry in New York City and, Joe said with some pride, earned nearly a million dollar a year at his peak. That peak, it turned out, had been some years earlier.

By Joe's senior year, his father was downsized and was out of a job. In his late 40s, he felt that he had limited prospects in the financial world. Though the family had maintained a life of privilege in appearance, Joe came to learn that their actual financial picture was rather grim. They had little in the way of liquid savings, and there was no way they would be able to pay the mortgage on their large home. What's more, they did not see how they would be able to send Joe to the very expensive private university that he planned on attending. They encouraged Joe to apply to a local state school and commute. They had a little savings left, but loans would still be needed. They were close to the end of the school year, so they would ride things out for a couple of months so that Joe could finish school with his class and graduate. But over the summer they would need to move.

Joe told none of his friends about what was happening. In fact, he didn't talk about it with anyone. Conversations with friends about parties and girls and the undoubted success that awaited them at college continued. But in the middle of July, Joe's family did move to a middle-class town not too far away where they rented a small house. Joe's parents thought it would be best to be near their old town. This way, Joe could still hang out with his friends and enjoy the summer. In Joe's mind, however, he would have preferred that the "dump of a house" that they rented be on the other side of the country, or somewhere in the middle of nowhere.

As I listened to Joe's story—told with a mix of bitterness, resentment, and sadness—I could hear the profound losses Joe had sustained and how they had crushed his youthful narcissism that, stoked by a life of privilege, had convinced him that the world was very much his oyster—his for the taking. Now, however, it felt that everything he wanted was beyond his reach. All these years later, it was hard to remember what that kind of confidence felt like. His narrative had changed so radically, and the story he told himself now was one of self-doubt and an uncertain future—a story that lay at the roots of his depression and anxiety.

Joe and I worked together for some time and managed to make some progress with his symptoms. His defenses against mourning his losses, however, were quite strong. Addressing the painful changes he experienced to his narrative of self and the life he imagined for himself was very difficult for him. He told me one day that he was feeling better and that he wanted to take a break from therapy. I talked with Joe about what more I believed we could accomplish together and encouraged him to come back to therapy, but I didn't see him again after that.

Grief Work in Clinical Practice: A Narrative Perspective

Throughout this chapter we have looked through a narrative lens at the many dynamics of grief and loss, and I have shared with you a number of vignettes illustrating a narrative approach. Let's turn now to something of a summary of this way of being with grief as well as some of the tools that may assist our clients on the journey. At its most elemental, I want to suggest that a narrative approach to grief and loss entails walking with and at times guiding our bereaved clients in the process of meaning making (Neimeyer, 2016a). Quite recently, I met a client for the first time. He had been through a gut-wrenching loss that left him feeling hollow and immobilized. He was eager for someone to help him, but at the same time could not imagine what kind of help there might be that could rescue him from the pain he was feeling. I told him, gently, some things I have said to others in similar positions, not because they are some sort of standard response, but because I genuinely believe they are true.

> "I think on some level when we are in the midst of what feels like a nightmare, we fantasize about turning back the clock or, for that matter, fast forwarding, anything to get back to that person we were and just how we felt before grief struck. Anything but how we feel now in the midst of grief. But the truth is we are never going to get to a place where this terrible loss and the pain you feel hasn't happened. It is a part of you now, a part of your story. And so the goal can't be to undo. The goal has to be to integrate, to find a way for this terribly painful experience to have its place in the overall story of you and your life, and then to continue living from there. And we'll do that together over time. I'll listen. You'll tell me the story. You'll work at making some sense of it, and I'll help you. And that sense – that meaning is going to change over time. But as we go along, I trust you'll find that you are discovering more and more of yourself, and feeling like yourself again. Not who you were then (though you may gain some new insight about that). But who you are now."

So the heart of this grief work is accompaniment and careful listening, trusting that the human spirit has a nearly indomitable way of bouncing back and finding meaning. This doesn't mean that we don't come through the process with some scars, but scars are a sign of healing and an assurance of survival. Perhaps some of you have read the novel *All the Pretty Horses* by Cormac McCarthy (1993). Though the novel as a whole is beautifully written, there was one line that gave me pause and made me reach for my pen. It is the only sentence I underlined in the book. "Scars have the strange power to remind us that our past is real" (p. 135). Scars tell a story. If you have any yourself (at least visible ones), you have probably been asked a time or two to tell the story of how you got them. I think the narratives of our grief and loss come to fit into our larger story in the same way. They stand out, and in coming to be they have often taken a toll on us. But they are part of who we are. They remind us that our past is real and they speak to our survival.

Along the way, there are various resources that our clients can make use of and that we can suggest to them. A spiritual or faith perspective is consistently noted in the literature as a tool in the process of renegotiating or finding meaning in the wake of loss (Burke & Neimeyer, 2014; Burke, Neimeyer, Young, Bonin, & Davis, 2014). This is true of a wide variety of faith traditions (Chatterjee, 2007; Kristiansen, Younis, Hassani, & Sheikh, 2016; McLellan, 2015; Neimeyer & Young-Eisendrath, 2015; Rubin, 2015). In this book, we have reflected on it as a source of ultimate meaning. Additionally, various creative forms of self-expression may be useful to a bereaved client. These might include things like directed journaling (Lichtenthal & Neimeyer, 2012), poetry, visual arts, dance, and music. Even from a narrative perspective, these latter media may be valuable in helping clients get to the emotional center of their experience when they do not have words. There is even evidence that Shakespeare may have used art as a way of expressing and coping with his grief, writing Hamlet following his son's death in 1596 and his father's death in 1601 (Dreher, 2016).

Finally, let me mention how important it is for the clinician to understand and process their own story of grief and loss in order to practice effectively with clients in this area. That doesn't mean that we need to be perfect of course. However, to the extent that we are not in touch with our own experience of loss and all that has gone into shaping our own narrative about grief, we risk doing an injustice to vulnerable clients who need us to sit with them, listen to them, and help them to make meaning out of some of the most painful experiences life can bring us.

Case Example

When Monique called to make an appointment she said that she had been referred by a local hospital. She didn't want to get into much detail on the phone. She said it was hard to talk just then. But she did want the first available appointment, and she agreed to an opening I had the following afternoon. When I greeted her in the waiting room the next day, she presented as a well-dressed, poised young professional. She was polite but reserved, an African-American woman in her early 30s. As we settled in, I asked her to tell me about the reason she was seeking therapy.

She spoke softly, almost in a hushed tone. She made little eye contact, either looking down to her lap or out the window. She got my number from a chaplain at the hospital, she said. She met him 2 weeks earlier when she was there. He had called to check on her as a follow-up. When he asked how she was doing, she said fine, thank you. But then she broke down in tears and told the chaplain that, in fact, she was not fine at all. She was having a hard time sleeping; she had no appetite. She could barely concentrate at work. Though Monique was telling me about symptoms that were certainly concerning, I was still unclear about what had brought this on. "Why was it, Monique, that you were at the hospital?"

"My husband died." She looked as if she herself did not believe the words that were coming out of her mouth. She continued. "It was a couple of weekends ago. Saturday morning. We were just hanging out. I had talked to my mother on the phone for a bit. I paid some bills. Jeff was in the living room playing video games … God, he loved that X-Box! We argued about it some times. I asked him why a grown man needed to spend so much time playing video games. 'That's how I relax,' he would say. 'Be glad I'm not out carrying on with my friends!' I suppose he was right actually."

"We talked about the plans for the day. Nothing much. We thought about maybe doing some shopping that afternoon. I wanted new bedroom furniture. He said maybe he'd go. We were supposed to meet friends for dinner that night. After lunch he said he didn't feel well. He had a headache, and wanted to take a nap, so I went out to run some errands. When I got back a couple of hours later he was still sleeping. I woke him to remind him about our dinner plans, but he said he didn't think he could go. He really didn't feel well. His body was aching. He had a high fever. He said he felt weak. I gave him some medicine for the fever and told him to lie back down. I called our friends to cancel for that night."

"And what a night it was! He couldn't sleep. The fever wasn't coming down. He was miserable. We thought it must be some kind of flu. I remember I was freaked out thinking I was going to catch it from him. Things just kept getting worse. So about 4:00 am Sunday, I said let's go to the emergency room. They have to be able to give you something stronger for this. When we got to the hospital they took his blood and started running all these tests. I remember thinking that it all seemed a bit overdone. They were probably just trying to make more money off the insurance. I honestly thought they were just going to write a couple of prescriptions and send us on our way. About an hour later a doctor came back with test results. I remember him looking at my husband and saying, 'Jeff, you're a very sick man. Let me explain what we're going to try.' 'Try.' I think that was the word that first made me panic. What did he mean, try? The doctor said that Jeff had some sort of infection – I forget what you call it – that had spread through his whole system. It was very aggressive and fast moving. They were transferring him to the I.C.U. They would try I.V. antibiotics, and some other things. He rattled off all these names. I didn't understand what he was talking about. He seemed nervous himself."

"And the look on Jeff's face ... He looked terrified. I couldn't believe how bad he looked. He was weak, ashy, sweating ... But his eyes were so wide. He looked so scared. I held his hand. It was hot and damp. And he was just holding onto me as hard as he could. A couple of minutes later, they were moving us to I.C.U. When we got there they asked me to wait outside. But the walls were glass so I could see. There had to be five people working on him. I don't even know what they were all doing. When they let me back in he was hooked up to all these monitors and I think three different I.V.'s ...."

"They tried really hard. I know they did. But that afternoon he died. It was 2:37. He lost consciousness towards the end. He was so scared." Monique wept. She was spent.

Monique returned to where she began. In the 2 weeks since Jeff's death she was having a hard time sleeping. She couldn't stand being alone in the apartment, getting into their bed. She tried sleeping on the couch, but it was just so hard to relax. She had no appetite even though everyone was telling her that she had to eat. She had gone back to work the previous week. Her boss was very nice and asked her if it was too soon, if she needed more time. No, she insisted, she had to get back to things. There was work waiting that needed to get done. Anyway, it would be a good distraction for her. She had stared at the walls in her apartment for long enough. The problem was at work she was doing little more than staring into empty space. She felt lost, confused, and trapped.

She had supports around her, including her and Jeff's families. They were all heart-broken, of course. When they were sent up to the I.C.U., Monique called Jeff's parents and they had come to the hospital. So did Monique's parents and a small group of their closest friends. Everyone was being very supportive, but she knew she needed something more. When the chaplain called from the hospital and suggested seeing someone for grief counseling, she knew he was right. Monique said that she felt comfortable talking with me and we agreed to meet once a week.

As the work of therapy got under way, I learned a lot more about Monique and Jeff and the backstory that set the context for Monique's experience of grief. She was able to identify fairly easily the feelings of ambivalence she was having. It turned out that she and Jeff were having problems. They had only been married 2 years, but there was a lot of arguing. She would get after him to step up and be more responsible, and get off the video games. He worked a good job and was responsible in that way, but that was it. He didn't help in any way around the house. He never wanted to go anywhere or do anything. For his part, she said, Jeff would get frustrated at times, angry really, and yell at her to get off his back. He said it felt like nothing was ever good enough for her.

They had actually talked about getting divorced. But just about a month earlier, they had had a good talk. She felt that they hadn't communicated that well since they first started dating. They agreed that they both really wanted to try to make it work, and had both made some changes. He was trying to be more involved and to do more around the house. He went grocery shopping a couple of times. He agreed to go out with friends. That's what they were supposed to do the night he got sick. She was trying to change too. She knew that she could be critical, and that it could come across as really harsh. So she was trying to soften that edge. She told herself that when she got frustrated with something, she should take a minute and breathe. She should think about what she wanted to say and how she wanted to say it. They were both trying to make it work. She didn't know if it would have worked but at least they were trying.

"The thing of it is," Monique said, "No one knew. No one knew that we were having problems, not my family, not his family. I only told my very best friend. Jeff said he didn't talk to his friends like that, so he didn't tell anyone at all. We thought it was best not to get the families involved. You know everyone's got an opinion. Everybody's got to get into everybody else's business. So we kept it to ourselves. It was our business. I only even talked to my best friend because I was trying to decide if I should leave him. That was before we decided to try to make things better."

I asked Monique if people not knowing about their marital problems was impacting her grief. She said it was, quite a bit. "Everybody is talking about Jeff and me as if we were this fairytale couple, so wonderful together, so in love. It's like we're characters in some romance novel, and it's all so tragic. I'm the princess weeping over my lost prince or something. And that's just it, it *is* tragic. It's terrible. But at the same time everyone's telling me about what they *imagine* I'm feeling, no one really *knows* what I'm feeling. It's like I'm trying to deal with what I'm feeling, but at the same time I have to deal with all these expectations everybody has. It all just feels kind of surreal. Hell, a month ago I was ready to kick Jeff out; now he's gone forever. I loved him. I truly did. But I'm not 100% sure he knew that. This is what I sit on the couch thinking about in the middle of the night. Can you believe it? Did he know I loved him? Did he really love me? I know he did."

Monique really was grieving. She wanted to make sure I understood that, and I did. Yes, they had had problems, but Monique loved her husband and everything about his death had turned her life upside down. It came out of nowhere. How could an infection spread that fast? And with all the medicines they have, why couldn't they save him? They needed more time; they had so much more to do and to say. Monique talked about mourning the loss of her dreams for herself and them as a couple. There had been a lot of mourning lately. She was mourning the happiness she felt when she first fell in love with Jeff and when they first got married. She was mourning the dream she had of their life together and what it would be like. She was mourning the children that they always assumed they would have. That had been the story of her life—the story of her future—and now she didn't know what direction that story would take. Every day was filled with sadness, and fear, and confusion.

She and Jeff were both religious people. They were Baptists. She said that she prayed every day that God would show her a way through her grief, and help her understand and know what to do next, and she prayed for Jeff. "How long am I going to feel this way," she asked one day in session. We had been working together about a month. "There's no way for either of us to know that exactly," I answered. "Grief isn't like an on/off switch, is it? It isn't like we just wake up one day and it's gone. It's more about how we change over time. So, I can't really tell you how long you'll feel the way you do. But I can make you one promise." "What's that," she asked.

"That you won't feel this way for ever. I don't know exactly how it's going to happen. But you will change; you will feel different. In fact, I'll bet that if you and I talk a year from now, whether we're still working together or we just touch base on the phone, you'll tell me that you feel different. I don't know what it will feel like or what will be going on in your life. But it will be different than this." "Ok," she said. "Let's hope."

Monique and I kept working with her grief, exploring the narrative of her life, her marriage to Jeff, his death, and more. Her storytelling in session over time came to include more about her life in the present and her thoughts about the future. We still talked about Jeff to be sure. Monique told me about everything from how they met and their courtship to the wedding and honeymoon, and the beginnings of their life together. And of course, we talked about his death—the events surrounding it and all that it meant for her. The quality of Monique's storytelling shifted gradually over time. Her thoughts about Jeff came to be a greater mix of sad and happy or even neutral. She still felt deeply sad; she cried at some point, even for a few minutes, most days. But it was less than before. She had more energy than before and was sleeping and eating better.

As the first anniversary of Jeff's death approached, Monique told me that she was feeling increasingly anxious. She worried about how she would feel on the day. Would the memories be too intense, overwhelming? She had never visited Jeff's grave. She hadn't been able to bring herself to do it, she said. But she had plans to go to the cemetery that day with Jeff's mother. I encouraged Monique to talk about the thoughts and fantasies she was having about that first anniversary and its meaning.

We talked about what it meant for her life both then and now. I also worked with her on ways to manage the anxiety she was feeling.

The anniversary itself and Monique's visit to the cemetery fell in the middle of the week between our sessions. We continued to explore her sense of anxious anticipation about this part of the story and what it might mean to her. I told her that even though we would not be meeting on the anniversary itself, I understood what a significant day it was for her on so many levels. I encouraged her to call me if she needed or wanted to after she visited the cemetery with her mother-in-law. She did just that. Monique said that the visit went "fine." She talked with Jeff, and told him that no matter what they had been through, she loved him. She always had. She cried, of course, and so did Jeff's mother. The two women prayed together and read from Scripture. They even sang a hymn, the same one as at Jeff's funeral—his favorite. Afterwards, they went out to lunch and she drove her mother-in-law home. It went fine—more than fine actually.

I assured Monique that I had been thinking of her that day, and was glad to hear that the visit had gone well. It was an important day for her. We confirmed our appointment for the following week and were about to hang up when Monique said,

"Oh, one more thing I wanted to say."
"What's that?"
"You remember when I first started coming to see you, I asked how long I was going to feel the way I was?"
"Sure. I remember."
"You made me a promise that day. You said that if we talked at the end of the year, you didn't know how I would be feeling but that it would be different – that I wouldn't be in the same place."
"I remember that too."
"Well, I thought a lot about that today, and you were right. It is different. I'm different. Life is different. It's not perfect, but it's not as it was ... Thanks."

Monique and I terminated therapy a few weeks later.

Questions and Activities for Discussion and Further Reflection

1. Reflect on your own experience of grief and loss. How has it contributed to your story of self, life, and the world? If you have not had much personal experience in this area, what have you understood through your relationship to others who have?
2. Consider the ways in which your own narrative about grief and loss has been shaped by the cultures and social groups to which you belong. Have a class discussion in which these social narratives are shared, compared, and contrasted.
3. Have you had the experience of sitting with a grieving client? (Note that this is different from being with a friend or family member.) What was it like for you to be in that emotional space with them? How did you handle that? How did it differ from coping with grief and loss in your personal life?
4. Throughout the chapter, I review a number of different kinds of loss both involving and not involving actual death. What other varieties of loss can you think of that might be the cause of grief for your clients? Choose one and do a literature search to find one or two articles, books, or chapters on this kind of loss. Review that material in order to learn more about it. Consider sharing your findings with your class.

5. Using one or more of the clinical vignettes in this chapter, role-play a session in which you explore with the client the narrative of their loss and the meaning they make of it. Tune into the story they are telling about their grief. Have other students observe, and then share thoughts and impressions. Focus not only on what was said, but also on the experience of being present to a grieving client.
6. Visit the website for the American Foundation for Suicide Prevention (www.afsp.org). Look at the resources they offer not only for suicide prevention, but also for the support of survivors. Discuss what you find as a class. Consider participating as a group in an AFSP walk or other event to offer your support to others.
7. Read *The Year of Magical Thinking*, by Joan Didion, *A Grief Observed* by C.S. Lewis, *Option B: Facing Adversity, Building Resilience, and Finding Joy* by Sheryl Sandberg and Adam Grant, or another first-person account of the lived reality of grief and loss. What do you learn from their narrative about the nature of that experience and the meaning they have made of it? How might that be useful to you in your work with clients?

References

Aldrich, H., & Kallivayalil, D. (2016). Traumatic grief after homicide: Intersections of individual and community loss. *Illness, Crisis, & Loss, 24*(1), 15–33. https://doi.org/10.1177/1054137315587630

Alves, D., Fernández-Navarro, P., Ribeiro, A. P., Ribeiro, E., Sousa, I., & Gonçalves, M. M. (2016). Ambivalence in grief therapy: The interplay between change and self-stability. *Death Studies, 40*(2), 129–138. https://doi.org/10.1080/07481187.2015.1102177

Baddeley, J., & Singer, J. A. (2010). A loss in the family: Silence, memory, and narrative identity after bereavement. *Memory, 18*(2), 198–207. https://doi.org/10.1080/09658210903143858

Bonanno, G. A. (2009). *The other side of sadness*. New York: Basic Books.

Bonanno, G. A., Westphal, M., & Mancini, A. D. (2011). Resilience to loss and potential trauma. *Annual Review of Clinical Psychology, 7*, 511–535.

Boss, P. (1999). *Ambiguous loss: Learning to live with unresolved grief*. Cambridge, MA: Harvard University Press.

Boss, P. (2010). The trauma and complicated grief of ambiguous loss. *Pastoral Psychology, 59*(2), 137–145. https://doi.org/10.1007/s11089-009-0264-0

Bruner, J. (1986). *Actual minds, possible worlds*. Cambridge, MA: Harvard University Press.

Bruner, J. (1987). Life as narrative. *Social Research, 54*, 11–32.

Bruner, J. (1990). *Acts of meaning*. Cambridge, MA: Harvard University Press.

Burke, L. A., & Neimeyer, R. A. (2014). Complicated spiritual grief I: Relation to complicated grief symptomatology following violent death bereavement. *Death Studies, 38*(4), 259–267. https://doi.org/10.1080/07481187.2013.829372

Burke, L. A., Neimeyer, R. A., Young, A. J., Bonin, E. P., & Davis, N. L. (2014). Complicated spiritual grief II: A deductive inquiry following the loss of a loved one. *Death Studies, 38*(4), 268–281. https://doi.org/10.1080/07481187.2013.829373

Butler, R. N. (1963). The life review: An interpretation of reminiscence in the aged. *Psychiatry, 26*, 65–76.

Chatterjee, S. C. (2007). Spiritual interventions in grief resolution: A personal narrative. *Illness, Crisis, & Loss, 15*(2), 113–124.

Clifton, S. (2014). Grieving my broken body: An autoethnographic account of spinal cord injury as an experience of grief. *Disability and Rehabilitation, 36*(21), 1823–1829. https://doi.org/10.3109/09638288.2013.872202

Collis, M. (2007). 'Mourning the loss' or 'no regrets': Exploring women's emotional responses to hysterectomy. In J. Davidson, L. Bondi, & M. Smith (Eds.), *Emotional geographies*. New York: Routledge.

Cornell, W. F. (2014). Grief, mourning, and meaning: In a personal voice. *Transactional Analysis Journal, 44*(4), 302–310. https://doi.org/10.1177/0362153714559921

Crossley, M. L. (2000). Narrative psychology, trauma and the study of self/identity. *Theory & Psychology, 10*(4), 527–546.

Crossley, M. L. (2003). Formulating narrative psychology: The limitations of contemporary social constructionism. *Narrative Inquiry, 13*(2), 287–300.

Currier, J. M., & Neimeyer, R. A. (2007). Fragmented stories: The narrative integration of violent loss. In E. K. Rynearson (Ed.), *Violent death: Resilience and intervention beyond the crisis* (pp. 85–100). New York: Routledge.

Didion, J. (2006a). *We tell ourselves stories in order to live: Collected nonfiction*. New York: Everyman's Library—Knopf.

Didion, J. (2006b). *The year of magical thinking*. New York: Vintage Books.

Doka, K. (Ed.). (2002). *Disenfranchised grief*. Champaign, IL: Research Press.

Dreher, D. E. (2016). To tell my story: Grief and self-disclosure in Hamlet. *Illness, Crisis, & Loss, 24*(1), 3–14.

Fernadez, R., Harris, D., & Leschied, A. (2011). Understanding grief following pregnancy loss: A retrospective analysis regarding women's coping responses. *Illness, Crisis, & Loss, 19*(2), 143–163. https://doi.org/10.2190/IL.19.2.d

Foster, R. P. (1998). *The power of language in the clinical process: Assessing and treating the bilingual person*. New York: Jason Aronson.

Freud, S. (1917/1957). Mourning and melancholia. In J. Strachey (Ed.), *The complete psychological works of Sigmund Freud*. London: Hogarth Press.

Gillespie, P. (2017). This is what clinical death looks like. *Illness, Crisis, & Loss, 25*(2), 127–149.

Goldstein, E. (2005). *When the bubble bursts: Clinical perspectives on midlife issues*. Hillsdale, NJ: Analytic Press.

Horowitz, A. V., & Wakefield, J. C. (2007). *The loss of sadness: How psychiatry transformed normal sadness into a depressive disorder*. New York: Oxford University Press.

Janoff-Bulman, R. (1992). *Shattered assumptions: Towards a new psychology of trauma*. New York: Free Press.

Janoff-Bulman, R. (2006). Schema-change perspectives on posttraumatic growth. In L. G. Calhoun & R. G. Tedeschi (Eds.), *Handbook of posttraumatic growth: Research and practice* (pp. 81–99). New York: Lawrence Erlbaum Associates.

Janoff-Bulman, R., & Frantz, C. M. (1997). The impact of trauma on meaning: From meaningless world to meaningful life. In M. Power & C. R. Brewin (Eds.), *The transformation of meaning in psychological therapies* (pp. 91–106). New York: Wiley.

Jones, S. L. (2015). The psychological miscarriage: An exploration of women's experience of miscarriage in the light of Winnicott's 'primary maternal preoccupation', the process of grief according to Bowlby and Parkes, and Klein's theory of mourning. *British Journal of Psychotherapy, 31*(4), 433–447. https://doi.org/10.1111/bjp.12172

Kitch, C. (2003). Mourning in America: Ritual, redemption, and recovery in new narrative after September 11. *Journalism Studies, 4*(2), 213–224.

Kristiansen, M., Younis, T., Hassani, A., & Sheikh, A. (2016). Experiencing loss: A Muslim widow's bereavement narrative. *Journal of Religion and Health, 55*(1), 226–240. https://doi.org/10.1007/s10943-015-0058-x

Kubler-Ross, E. (1969). *On death and dying*. New York: MacMillan.

Lewis, C. S. (1961). *A grief observed*. New York: Harper Collins.

Lichtenthal, W. G., & Neimeyer, R. A. (2012). Directed journaling to facilitate meaning making. In R. A. Neimeyer (Ed.), *Techniques of grief therapy* (pp. 165–168). New York: Routledge.

Lichtenthal, W. G., Neimeyer, R. A., Currier, J. M., Roberts, K., & Jordan, N. (2013). Cause of death and the quest for meaning after the loss of a child. *Death Studies, 37*(4), 311–342. https://doi.org/10.1080/07481187.2012.673533

Lindemann, E. (1944). Symptomatology and management of acute grief. *American Journal of Psychiatry, 101*, 141–148.

Maercker, A., Brewin, C. R., Bryant, R. A., Cloitre, M., Reed, G. M., van Ommeren, M., … Saxena, S. (2013). Proposals for mental disorders specifically associated with stress in the International Classification of Diseases-11. *The Lancet, 381*(9878), 1683–1685. https://doi.org/10.1016/S0140-6736(12)62191-6

Maercker, A., & Lalor, J. (2012). Diagnostic and clinical considerations in prolonged grief disorder. *Dialogues in Clinical Neuroscience, 14*, 167–176.

McCarthy, C. (1993). *All the pretty horses*. New York: Vintage Books.

McCreight, B. S. (2004). A grief ignored: Narratives of pregnancy loss from a male perspective. *Sociology of Health & Illness, 26*(3), 326–350. https://doi.org/10.1111/j.1467-9566.2004.00393.x

McCreight, B. S. (2008). Perinatal loss: A qualitative study in Northern Ireland. *Omega, 57*(1), 1–19. https://doi.org/10.2190/OM.57.1.a

McGoldrick, M. (2004). Gender and mourning. In F. Walsh & M. McGoldrick (Eds.), *Living beyond loss: Death in the family* (pp. 99–118). New York, NY: W. W. Norton.

McLellan, J. (2015). Religious responses to bereavement, grief, and loss among refugees. *Journal of Loss and Trauma, 20*(2), 131–138. https://doi.org/10.1080/15325024.2013.833807

Neimeyer, R. A. (2001a). The language of loss: Grief therapy as a process of meaning reconstruction. In R. A. Neimeyer (Ed.), *Meaning reconstruction and the experience of loss* (pp. 261–292). Washington, DC: American Psychological Association.

Neimeyer, R. A. (2004). Fostering posttraumatic growth: A narrative contribution. *Psychological Inquiry, 15*, 53–59.

Neimeyer, R. A. (2005). Tragedy and transformation: Meaning reconstruction in the wake of traumatic loss. In S. Heilman (Ed.), *Death, bereavement, and mourning*. New Brunswick, NJ: Transaction Publishers.

Neimeyer, R. A. (2006). Re-storying loss: Fostering growth in the posttraumatic narrative. In L. G. Calhoun & R. G. Tedeschi (Eds.), *Handbook of posttraumatic growth: Research and pracice* (pp. 68–80). New York: Lawrence Erlbaum Associates.

Neimeyer, R. A. (2016a). Helping clients find meaning in grief and loss. In M. Cooper & W. Dryden (Eds.), *The handbook of pluralistic counseling and psychotherapy* (pp. 211–222). Thousand Oaks, CA: Sage.

Neimeyer, R. A. (2016b). You were born, still: The search for meaning in perinatal loss. In K. Doka & A. Tucci (Eds.), *Managing conflict, finding meaning*. Washington, DC: Hospice Foundation of America.

Neimeyer, R. A. (Ed.). (2001b). *Meaning reconstruction and the experience of loss*. Washington, DC: American Psychological Association.

Neimeyer, R. A., & Harris, D. (2016). Bereavement and grief. In H. S. Friedman (Ed.), *Encyclopedia of mental health* (2nd ed., pp. 163–169). Waltham, MA: Academic Press.

Neimeyer, R. A., Klass, D., & Dennis, M. R. (2014). A social constructionist account of grief: Loss and the narration of meaning. *Death Studies, 38*(8), 485–498. https://doi.org/10.1080/07481187.2014.913454

Neimeyer, R. A., & Young-Eisendrath, P. (2015). Assessing a Buddhist treatment for bereavement and loss: The Mustard Seed Project. *Death Studies, 39*(5), 263–273. https://doi.org/10.1080/07481187.2014.937973

Park, C. L., & Folkman, S. (1997). Meaning in the context of stress and coping. *Review of General Psychology, 1*(2), 115–144.

Peri, T., Hasson-Ohayon, I., Garber, S., Tuval-Mashiach, R., & Boelen, P. A. (2016). Narrative reconstruction therapy for prolonged grief disorder—Rationale and case study. *European Journal of Psychotraumatology, 7*, 1–11.

Piot-Ziegler, C., Sassi, M. L., Raffoul, W., & Delaloye, J. F. (2010). Mastectomy, body deconstruction, and impact on identity: A qualitative study. *British Journal of Health Psychology, 15*(3), 479–510. https://doi.org/10.1348/135910709X472174

Price, J. E., & Jones, A. M. (2015). Living through the life-altering loss of a child: A narrative review. *Issues in Comprehensive Pediatric Nursing, 38*(3), 222–240. https://doi.org/10.3109/01460862.2015.1045102

Pritchard, T. R., & Buckle, J. L. (2017). Meaning-making after partner suicide: A narrative exploration using the meaning of loss codebook. *Death Studies*. https://doi.org/10.1080/07481187.2017.1334007

Rubin, S. S. (1999). The two-track model of bereavement: Overview, retrospect and prospect. *Death Studies, 23*, 681–714.

Rubin, S. S. (2015). Loss and mourning in the Jewish tradition. *Omega, 70*(1), 79–98. https://doi.org/10.2190/OM.70.1.h

Sands, D. C., Jordan, J. R., & Neimeyer, R. A. (2010). The meanings of suicide: A narrative approach to healing. In J. R. Jordan & J. L. MacIntosh (Eds.), *Grief after suicide* (pp. 249–281). New York: Routledge.

Sawicka, M. (2016). Searching for a narrative of loss: Interactional ordering of ambiguous grief. *Symbolic Interaction, 40*(2) 229–246. https://doi.org/10.1002/symb.270

Stikkelbroek, Y., Bodden, D. H. M., Reitz, E., Vollerbergh, W. A. M., & van Baar, A. L. (2016). Mental health of adolescents before and after the death of a parent or sibling. *European Child & Adolescent Psychiatry, 25*(1), 49–59.

Stroebe, M., & Schut, H. (2010). The dual process model of coping with bereavement. A decade on. *Omega, 61*, 273–289.

Sveen, J., Eilegard, A., Steineck, G., & Kreicbergs, U. (2014). They still grieve: A nationwide follow-up of young adults 2-9 years after losing a sibling to cancer. *Psycho-Oncology, 23*(6), 658–664. https://doi.org/10.1002/pon.3463

Tadel, P. M. (2014). Wading in the water: A case study approach to engaging more fully in the patient narrative. *Illness, Crisis, & Loss, 22*(1), 11–27.

Tan, J. S., Docherty, S. L., Barfield, R., & Brandon, D. H. (2012). Addressing parental bereavement support needs at the end of life for infants with complex chronic conditions. *Journal of Palliative Medicine, 15*(5), 579–584. https://doi.org/10.1089/jpm.2011.0357

Volkan, V., & Zintl, E. (1993). *Life after loss: The lessons of grief.* London: Karnac Books.

Walsh, F., & McGoldrick, M. (Eds.). (2004). *Living beyond loss: Death in the family.* New York: W. W. Norton.

Werner-Lin, A., & Moro, T. (2004). Unacknowledged and stigmatized losses. In F. Walsh & M. McGoldrick (Eds.), *Living beyond loss: Death in the family* (pp. 247–271). New York, NY: W. W. Norton.

Westerhof, G. J., & Bohlmeijer, E. T. (2014). Celebrating fifty years of research and applications in reminiscence and life review: State of the art and new directions. *Journal of Aging Studies, 29*, 107–114. https://doi.org/10.1016/j.jaging.2014.02.003

Worden, J. W. (1991). *Grief counseling and grief therapy: A handbook for the mental health practitioner* (2nd ed.). New York, NY: Springer.

Wright, P. M. (2016). Adult sibling bereavement: Influences, consequences, and interventions. *Illness, Crisis, & Loss, 24*(1), 34–45. https://doi.org/10.1177/1054137315587631

Chapter 8
Who I Am and Who I Want to Be: Narrative and the Evolving Self of the Social Worker in Clinical Practice

Guiding Questions

What made you want to become a social worker?
What kind of social worker do you want to be?
Who are your mentors and professional role models?
What does narrative have to say to us as social workers and clinicians about our roles and how we live them?
How do your values shape your vision of what it means to be a social worker and clinician?
What strategies will nourish your ongoing development as a social worker?

I can remember vividly the beginning of social work school. I was living in Westchester, New York, at the time. I took the Metro North train into Grand Central Station and then the subway down to 14th street. I was going to walk from there down to NYU. It was orientation day. I remember it was hot and humid, and had a pit in my stomach. Not just that, "Aw shucks, it's the first day of school" feeling of butterflies. It was more of a "Oh no, what have I gotten myself into?" kind of feeling. I was in my early 30s, and I had a sense that there had just been a little more change in my recent life than I frankly cared for. And now this. So I made a bargain with myself. I would go to orientation. It's one day; go in and sit there. What could it hurt? Just keep walking, I told myself. Clearly the day went fine—more than fine actually. It was great. I left interested, enthusiastic, and eager to start my classes. I share that story because it has always been a significant one in my narrative of becoming a social worker. There are lots more of course, some that come before, others that follow. We all have them.

This chapter is about you. It is about the story of how you came to be a social worker (or at least to want to be one) and what that means to you. I intend for this chapter to be different from the others in *Narrative Theory in Clinical Social Work Practice*. I would like to think of it more as a guided reflection. If you want to do this work, and do it well, I suggest that there are some things you need to know and others you need to wonder about, and likely come back to again over time. Like all narratives, the story that leads to the intersection of our personal and professional selves is a complex one. It is also one that is intimately connected to the way we do our work and the satisfaction we are able to find in it.

In Chapt. 1 I made the point that in clinical practice *you* are the instrument. The way we engage, listen, understand, and respond, with or without words, is processed through the only real tool of our trade—our self (Baldwin, 2013). We can apply to ourselves very readily the ancient dictum *know thyself*. For our purposes, however, perhaps we should say *know thy story*. Think of all you now know about social construction and narrative. Everything we have learned, all that life has taught us, the experiences we have had, whatever they may be, have all had a hand in shaping our story. That story has been elaborated from the social and cultural influences to which we have been exposed as well as the host of unique characteristics and forces that have shaped our personal environment and experiences. This is the narrative inheritance that we bring to the journey of becoming a social worker and to living that role with our clients and colleagues. So I'd like to offer some questions for your consideration. They are meant to help you get in touch with pieces of your story that have brought you to this point and that shape your vision of what your future might look like. Perhaps as you read and reflect you will think of other questions that are pertinent as you explore your own story. By all means, follow where they lead.

So, Why Do You Want to Be a Social Worker?

That is a question that we all have likely been asked at one point or another. Perhaps we had to write about it in an essay, or were asked it in an admissions interview. Maybe a relative or friend asked you at a holiday dinner or when you were just hanging out. Your answer at the time, even over time, may have been a more or less standard one (e.g., "I really want to help people."). You might have said it countless times and now it comes out automatically without even thinking about it, like a bedtime story that you memorized from sheer repetition but don't even listen to anymore. I would really like to encourage you to think about it though. If you are a student or if you are already out in the field, why do you want to be a social worker?

Some particular mix of life experiences brought you to this point. Let yourself wonder about what they were. Like an archaeologist at a dig, sift through the layers of the story. Your best insights might be very close to the surface, readily available. Or they might be deeper down. Be patient; you'll get there. This is what I referred to earlier as the intersection of your personal and professional selves. If you prefer, you could think of it as the weaving together of your personal and professional narratives. Here's one layer. Pay attention to the social narratives that are meaningful to you and that draw you to social work.

You might begin by asking yourself which social work values are most important to you. What are you passionate about? I have commonly found that when we are in touch with what excites or outrages us, we have tapped into the things we value most deeply. That kind of caring comes from some dimension of the personal story that brought us to the profession. So what is that for you? Perhaps someone taught you the importance of caring for the vulnerable, or to value justice. Who was that? How did they impact your life? Perhaps something you saw happening in the social environment filled you with indignation or interest, and made you want to get involved and do something? What was that? How did it move you?

On another level, it may be that something far more personal brought you to social work. I've had occasion to read quite a number of the essays that I referred to earlier: the ones that address "Why I want to be a social worker." I am always struck by the variety of personal experiences that have brought people to the profession. Often enough they are stories of pain and the overcoming of great adversity. This may involve struggles or divisions in one's family, a tragic loss, or a trauma that one has sustained. It may involve a significant medical illness, one's own or that of a loved one, or a personal or family battle with depression, anxiety, or addiction.

Typically, our stories involve some form of helping or being helped. We return again and again to the friends, family, and sometimes people we hardly even know, who told us that we were easy to talk to and that our presence or our words helped them. And we think of those who were there for us: the school social worker who was the only one who really seemed to listen to that child whose parents were getting divorced, the counselor who helped us find our way out of an addiction or an eating disorder, the therapist who really helped us to know that it was ok to feel what we were feeling, and that we could tell our story to another human being without the roof falling in as we had so long feared. These are deeply powerful, formative parts of our narrative that often inspire us to want to help others.

The now classic image that is used for this dynamic is that of the *wounded healer*. The metaphor speaks to the reality that, though we are professionally in a position through which we work to alleviate the suffering of others, we each carry with us the pain that is part of our own story. Though it is an ancient mythological archetype, the notion of the wounded healer was first applied to the person of the therapist by Jung (1963) who wrote that "only the wounded physician heals" (p. 134). Since Jung's initial articulation of this insight, an extensive literature has explored the ramifications of being a wounded healer in the work of psychotherapy (Jackson, 2001; Miller & Baldwin, 2013; Zerubavel & O'Dougherty-Wright, 2012).

The mixed bag of experience that brings us to the profession is often a perfectly fine way to begin, though there is more that is required. For one thing, it is essential that we be deeply in touch with that story and the way it motivates us. Just as I have been saying in different ways throughout this book, we need to understand the story we tell ourselves about who we are and what we are really doing in this work. Sometimes that story is quite apparent to us. However, sometimes it is buried much deeper. Somewhere deep down, we may be playing out the story that by helping our clients we will really be helping our mother or father, our sister or brother. By helping our clients we will be rescuing the friend who committed suicide and to whom we regret not having paid closer attention. We may even imagine that we will be saving ourselves by becoming the listener or healer that we so very much needed, but couldn't find.

To the extent that we are not in touch with that story, we run the risk not only of being sorely disappointed by our experience of the social work profession, but also of doing real harm to the clients who come to us for help. Thus, it is of great importance that the therapist become aware of his or her unconscious motivations for choosing this profession (Barnett, 2007; Farber, Manevich, Metzger, & Saypol, 2005). If we are consciously or unconsciously playing out the story of our own woundedness in our work, we are unavailable to truly attend to the story of our clients. We convince ourselves that we already know what the recovering addict is going to tell us; we've been there ourselves. We know depression so well that we implicitly understand what it is like to be our client and how they feel. To the degree that we filter what we take in from the client through our own particular set of limitations, we fail to tune into our client's actual narrative. These are dangerous blind spots that have no place in clinical practice. Most of the time, I believe it is possible for us to do enough work with our own narrative that we can be available in a helpful way to clients—though that may involve choosing not to work in certain fields of practice that hit too close to home. If I'm being honest, however, I also believe that there are times when the pain in our own story is so great that it is not productive, either for clients or ourselves, for us to take on the role of a professional helper.

It has been my experience that an invaluable outcome of good social work education is that it can disabuse us of the notion that our natural instincts and desire to be helpful are enough. Anyone who has gotten good at this work has learned some real-life lessons about what that takes, both in the classroom and in the field. And in this we find a great source of appropriate humility. I often raise for my students a question that is asked by people who feel leery of therapy and doubtful that the process could be of any use to them. "Why would I go talk to a therapist? I have friends and family; I can just talk to them. They really know me." If students are just beginning or haven't had occasion to give this some real thought, it can be a hard question to answer. My response goes back to something I discussed in Chap. 1 on the fundamental workings of narrative in clinical practice. The real issue that comes into play when we think about the value and uniqueness of therapy has to do with presence and listening.

Of course a person can talk to their family and friends about their concerns. Of course, your family and friends know you, at least to a certain extent. But if you've ever been cut off by a friend who wanted to be "helpful" and show you how much they understood by telling their own story that is just like yours (but not really), or by a relative who tried to tell you why your feelings were all wrong because they understood the situation and the people involved (possibly including even you) better than you do, then you might have some appreciation of the disciplined presence, and the finely honed, nonjudgmental listening skills of a good therapist. You might also appreciate the safety and containment of a therapeutic space where you can step aside from the routine of your daily life to pursue some understanding of yourself and your story. And if you've made any effort to develop those skills, you know just how much that demands. In short, this is what sets us apart from the concerned family member or friend who is well intentioned and might even be a pretty good listener. We are professionals who have usually invested an enormous amount of time in our personal and intellectual preparation for the work we do. And we are still working at it.

Study and Supervision in the Social Worker's Self-Narrative

This brings us two essential components of the developing narrative of a social worker: study and supervision. Whenever one embarks on a program of professional education, there are a couple of different tasks that are being undertaken simultaneously. One of these is the process of mastery of a body of information. In the world of social work this means a course of study that includes human behavior in the social environment, social work practice, social welfare policy, and social work research. The Council on Social Work Education sees to it that all accredited social work programs conform, at least in their broad outline, to a prescribed schema of academic preparation (Council on Social Work Education, 2015). Talk to any practicing social worker and they have taken courses in all these areas. Each school puts its own spin on the curriculum, as does each professor in their own way. That's what gives programs and classes their individual flavor. But we generally agree that if you want to be a social worker there are certain things you should know and know how to do.

I want to ask you to pause though and think about your academic social work education for a minute. If you are already out practicing in the field, think back on it. Ask yourself what stood out. Are there things you read that made a particular impression on you? Certain classes you took? Are there things you studied that you felt were a big waste of time? If you're a seasoned social worker, did that turn out to be true? The Latin root of the word education means to lead forth; education is meant to draw something out of you while it instills something in you. If social work schools do their job right, then you should leave at the end of your program with a very different understanding of the human person in the social environment than when you first walked through the front door. Think about it in this way: from generation to generation social work education is passing on a growing body of knowledge. That is a core part of our story.

But there is more to it than that. It's not only information. If we do our job right, you come out of social work school thinking, talking, and seeing the world like a social worker. We refer to this as professional socialization (Miller, 2013; Valutis, Rubin, & Bell, 2012). It is the adoption of the shared narrative of the profession. You're using terms like person-in-environment and biopsychosocial. You go out into the field with a deeper awareness of diversity and the dynamics of privilege. You tune into human behavior and its many meanings. You recognize the voices and instruments of oppression when you hear and see them, and you have some sense of what you can do about it. This whole process is about passing on to you the collective narrative that social workers have been building and sharing since the time of Jane Addams and Mary Richmond—the story of how we think, and of what we value.

Beyond the body of actual information then, there are real people who are the bearers and tellers of that story. They are theorists and researchers whose work you read and integrate, who offer you frames of reference like attachment, and systems, and ego functions and defenses. They teach you why correlation is not causation. They are professors who think out loud for you and have the privilege, every once in a while, of making an impression on you and shaping the way you think and see the world. It is an apprenticeship of sorts as we each get to follow in the footsteps of and learn from the ones who go before us. If you're lucky, you've had one or two who have made this kind of impression on you. I know I was very lucky in this way. I have suggested to students sometimes that we think of the voices of all these theorists and teachers like an invisible circle of advisors standing behind us as we work, helping us to tune into the meaning beneath the words and make sense of them, informing our listening and responding.

Outside the classroom, when we get into a field placement as students and then practice as professionals, there is supervision. This is a terribly important role in the initial and ongoing development of a social worker. Again, talk to any social worker and they will remember the best, and unfortunately the worst, supervisors they have had. These women and men stay with us because of the significance of what they do and represent in our professional life. Supervisors are the ones who teach us to write a treatment plan, progress notes, and a discharge plan. If they are really good though, they do something much more than that. They help us take the story of all that information and cumulative wisdom that is being passed onto us in the classroom, as well as the uniquely personal qualities that we bring to our work, and integrate them in the actual practice of our profession. I have written elsewhere of the particular role that supervision plays in helping us develop the use of self we spoke of earlier (McTighe, 2011). Whether you are a professional social worker who is supervising now, or a student who will almost certainly be asked to supervise in the future, I want to encourage you to take this seriously and remain mindful of the hand you have in the construction of your supervisee's narrative of their professional self. Take up the challenge of being just like the wonderful supervisor you had—or even wish you had.

With all this in mind, come back to the question with which we began. Why do you want to be a social worker? Dig deep. The answers to these questions, answers that will evolve over time, will take us a long way to understanding the nuances of our personal and professional social work narrative.

Considering Our Destinations

For now, let's turn our attention in a different direction. We have considered the pieces of our story that emerge from our personal and professional origins as social workers. Now let's focus on our destinations. What do you see yourself doing as a social worker and what do you imagine it will be like? If you are already practicing in the field, try to think back to what your earliest expectations were. Ask yourself how and to what extent your actual lived experience of the profession has measured up to those.

I have known a number of social workers who went to social work school convinced that all they wanted to do was be a school social worker or work in early child development. They were terribly disappointed and sometimes even angry when they found out that their first-year field placement would be in a nursing home. Today they are seasoned geriatric social workers who are in love with what they do. It comes down to a simple lesson, so simple in fact that we easily miss it. You only know what you know. There are people who knew they wanted to be accountants from the time they were 7 and counted up the take from their first lemonade stand, and that is fine. But narrative tells us that the future remains to be written, and that is an essential insight not only for career planning, but also for the nature of our clinical work.

When I was a student in Social Work Practice I, the course was team-taught by two women who were interesting, unconventional, and highly seasoned family therapists. That meant that the class was somewhat unconventional as well. I soon found that if you just went along for the ride and paid attention, the learning was tremendous. In one of the earliest class sessions we were told to divide ourselves into pairs, making sure to be with someone we didn't know. We were to interview each other and then introduce our partner to the class. That's standard enough fare for a practice class where you are learning basic interviewing skills, but there was a twist. We were given a question that we were supposed to think about and then discuss with our partner. The question was "What is it like for you *not* to know?" No explanation or elaboration. For some of us, it felt like we were participating in an ironic live experiment, since we weren't necessarily sure what the professors meant by the question.

As we settled into our interviews and discussion, and then reported out to the large group, it was remarkable what that simple question brought up for my classmates and me. It turns out that "not knowing" evoked for us some combination of anxiety, stress, curiosity, annoyance, confusion, resignation, nausea, and the occasional headache. We started to see that the implications of this simple exercise were rather profound. Our teachers helped us see further, introducing us to an aspect of practice that we were not yet able to anticipate on our own. You see, if you have a fantasy that you are going to be the fixer who takes the profession of social work by storm, conquering difficult problems left and right, you may find the real experience of clinical work rather challenging.

It turns out that a good deal of what we do in social work involves entering into the unknown. It is something we have to get used to. This is true of the profession itself when we are starting out, and it remains true in some ways of every professional transition we make. Each move to a new job, a new kind of responsibility, or a new role is a step into the unknown. For many of us, these leaps into the unknown are particularly anxiety provoking. In my own life, I have learned over the years to trust myself and my story enough to remind myself that taking that step isn't everything; it's just the next thing. It doesn't take away all anxiety since anxiety is a normal part of life. But it does help put the anxiety in its place and prevent it from stalling all forward movement. It allows our story to continue evolving.

This insight is not only true of our overall experience of the profession, however. It can actually shed a lot of light on the heart of what we do. Every time we meet a new client we are opening the door to someone new. In this way both of our stories advance individually and together. Consider that over the course of your social work career you might work with hundreds of individuals, couples, families, or groups that have some vey basic things in common. They might, for example, share a diagnosis of depression. Many might have endured trauma in some way or be mourning the loss of a loved one. The list could go on and on. But for whatever they have in common, every new client means an encounter with a narrative that is also new and unique, and the beginning of a new therapeutic relationship that will have its own character and meaning.

What's more, every session invites us to step into the unknown as we allow the story of that person to unfold and take shape through our encounter, and the intersecting narratives of client and therapist evolve right along with it. In my experience, even when we have known and worked with a client for years, each session is still new. This is true even if you are a therapist who works in a highly active and structured way with a planned agenda for each session. Not only are we not aware of what has transpired since the last session, but we also don't know what internal or relational processing has occurred or how the client's understanding of their own narrative of our work together has been interpreted. Certainly there are times when clients more or less "pick up where they left off." Often enough clients are eager to update us with the latest details of what they are going through. This kind of material can be quite important especially when our work is heavily focused on helping the client manage situations in their day-to-day life.

Simultaneously, however, that disciplined presence and listening that we bring to our work as professionals can help us tune in to the broader scope of meaning that is being related in their storytelling. This is the manifestation in the clinical situation of what I described in the previous chapters as the relationship between situational and global meaning (Park & Folkman, 1997), or micro- and macro-narratives (Neimeyer, 2004). We are in effect attending to two unfolding narratives at the same time. And while all of this is going on we are monitoring the pulse of our relationship with the client, trying to make the best use of our self in order to deepen our alliance and allow our work together to be as healing as possible. Though many of us have what is arguably a rather sedentary job, we are in a different way extremely active. The kind of attention we give and personal investment that we make in our work can make it exhausting. This brings us to our next point.

This Work Is Hard

As social workers and clinicians we will routinely be called upon to contain, interpret, and metabolize any number of stories that may be painful and even overwhelming. We will sit with feelings, memories, and experiences that clients bring to us in the hope that we can help them understand and integrate them into their narratives of self, life, and the world. We will encounter things on a regular basis that are new and different. Additionally, as we discussed earlier, the profession is continually advancing and it is our job to stay current. All this means a couple of things for us. First, you are never done getting to know yourself. There is always more to discover, more to understand. After all, you are an ever-evolving being. Beyond that though, I suspect you will find that the clients we work with over time have a way of tapping into our own developing narrative and drawing new things from us that have an impact on our work with them.

Second, you are never done learning. You may rejoice the day you get out of social work school and promise yourself that you are never going back to school again. But you must never stop learning and integrating that learning into your work. There are a number of tools we have at our disposal to help us accomplish this. First is good supervision. No matter how long we have been at this, we can always benefit from the wisdom and perspective of a good supervisor. Have you ever had the experience of watching a movie that you had seen many times with someone who has never seen it before? For all the times you may have seen that movie, someone watching it with new eyes can pick up things you never noticed before, or maybe once knew and had forgotten. Our clinical work can be very much like that. Sometimes we may be so close to it that it becomes hard to understand what is going on. A good supervisor can offer us that fresh perspective to listen to a case and give us feedback that might otherwise elude us.

As I discussed earlier, however, there is even more that a good supervisor can help us with. He or she can help us bring together the many strands of our story and weave them into a deeper and richer professional sense of self. That is an evolving tool that will serve us well throughout our career. In my own experience supervising social work students, I have had a number of supervisees who voiced their hopes for their own professional development. At the beginning of our relationship I have typically asked them to reflect on what gains they would like to make as a result of their field experience. What would they like to learn? How would they like to grow and be different by the end of their placement? This has commonly come around in some way to the issue of developing their professional sense of self. How are they to figure out how to pull everything together and make sense of it all? How are they to learn the skills of clinical practice in such a way that they can really make them their own?

Because our sense of self and our narrative as social workers is so intertwined with the story of our personal life and the social environments in which we have been formed, I believe that there is really no way to come to a mature professional identity except by becoming most fully who we are as individuals. The goal of supervision then is not to get you to think like me, practice like me, or see the world as I do. It is to help you become more fully you—to help you integrate your own narrative of what it means to be a social worker so that you are as available as possible for the work you do.

The second important tool is meaningful continuing education. It is easy enough to accumulate a patchwork of credits in whatever happens to be available and whatever is easiest. Some of them might even be free. But I want to encourage you to invest in your ongoing education for your clients' sake and your own as well. The ongoing development of your knowledge base and skills, particularly in whatever field of practice you are working in, will help you stay fresh and be effective. Stay in tune with the developing narrative of the profession. This fosters our own narrative of what it means to be a social worker and what is most important to us.

Third, do things that nourish your body, mind, and spirit. We now have an extensive literature that documents the real importance of investing in our own well-being if we are to continue doing this work (Skovholt & Trotter-Mathison, 2016). In our profession, the risks of burnout (Maslach, 2003; Schaufeli, Maslach, & Marek, 2017), compassion fatigue/secondary traumatic stress (Figley, 1995), vicarious trauma (Dunkley & Whelan, 2006; Pearlman & Mac Ian, 1995), and shared trauma (Saakvitne, 2002; Tosone, Nuttman-Shwartz, & Stephens, 2012) are real. Because of this, find whatever it is that is most restorative for you and commit some time and energy to it. Take a walk. Read a book—for leisure. Learn something new that has nothing to do with your work. Immerse yourself in some period of silence or meditation. Hold someone you love. All of these self-care activities are deeply important when you listen for a living, and expend your energy trying to help clients make sense of the story of their experience.

Lastly, pass it on. One of the best ways of staying in tune with your own story of what it means to be a social worker is to reflect on it and share it with someone else. Listen to a colleague, not just for the venting or complaining that we all probably need to do from time to time, but to gain a real understanding of their point of view. Supervise someone else; this may come in the form of peer supervision, which is often wonderful if we find the right colleagues to share with. Now or in the future, it may come by way of a more formal supervisory relationship. Give yourself to it thoughtfully, allowing yourself to be open to the narrative that is unfolding before you.

To be a social worker and a clinician is a privilege. It is a gift to be granted access to the most meaningful stories in the lives of those who seek our help, and to create with them a story of healing. Throughout this book we have reflected on the many ways in which narrative presents itself in our life and work, whether through our race and ethnicity, the traumas that have impacted us and from which we strive to rise up, the spirituality that sets the ultimate context for our living, the sexuality that grounds us in our bodies and draws us together, the strivings of the newest arrivals in our midst, or the ones we have lost and for whom we mourn. Remember to listen for the stories. They are all around us.

References

Baldwin, M. (2013). *The use of self in therapy* (3rd ed.). New York: Routledge.

Barnett, M. (2007). What brings you here? An exploration of the unconscious motivations of those who choose to train and work as psychotherapists and counselors. *Psychodynamic Practice, 13*, 257–274. https://doi.org/10.1080/14753630701455796

Council on Social Work Education. (2015). *2015 educational policy and accreditation standards for baccalaureate and master's social work programs*. Alexandria, VA: Council on Social Work Education.

Dunkley, J., & Whelan, T. A. (2006). Vicarious traumatization: Current status and future directions. *British Journal of Guidance and Counselling, 43*(1), 107–116.

Farber, B. A., Manevich, I., Metzger, J., & Saypol, E. (2005). Choosing psychotherapy as a career: Why did we cross that road? *Journal of Clinical Psychology/In Session, 61*(8), 1009–1031.

Figley, C. R. (Ed.). (1995). *Compassion fatigue: Coping with secondary traumatic stress disorder in those who treat the traumatized*. New York: Brunner-Routledge.

Jackson, S. W. (2001). The wounded healer. *Bulletin of the History of Medicine, 75*(1), 1–36. https://doi.org/10.1353/bhm.2001.0025

Jung, C. G. (1963). *Memories, dreams, reflections*. New York: Pantheon Books.

Maslach, C. (2003). *Burnout: The cost of caring*. Los Altos, CA: Malor Books.

McTighe, J. P. (2011). Teaching the use of self through the process of clinical supervision. *Clinical Social Work Journal, 39*(3), 301–307. https://doi.org/10.1007/s10615-010-0304-3

Miller, G. D., & Baldwin, D. C. (2013). The implications of the wounded-healer archetype for the use of self in psychotherapy. In M. Baldwin (Ed.), *The use of self in therapy* (3rd ed., pp. 81–96). New York: Routledge.

Miller, S. E. (2013). Professional socialization: A bridge between the explicit and implicit curricula. *Journal of Social Work Education, 49*(3), 368–386.

Neimeyer, R. A. (2004). Fostering posttraumatic growth: A narrative contribution. *Psychological Inquiry, 15*(1), 53–59.

Park, C. L., & Folkman, S. (1997). Meaning in the context of stress and coping. *Review of General Psychology, 1*(2), 115–144.

Pearlman, L. A., & Mac Ian, P. S. (1995). Vicarious traumatization: An empirical study of the effects of trauma work on trauma therapists. *Professional Psychology: Research and Practice, 26*(6), 558–565.

Saakvitne, K. W. (2002). Shared trauma: The therapist's increased vulnerability. *Psychoanalytic Dialogues, 12*(3), 443–449.

Schaufeli, W. B., Maslach, C., & Marek, T. (Eds.). (2017). *Professional burnout: Recent developments in theory and research* (3rd ed.). New York: Routledge.

Skovholt, T. M., & Trotter-Mathison, M. (2016). *The resilient practitioner: Burnout and compassion fatigue prevention and self-care strategies for the helping professions* (3rd ed.). New York: Routledge.

Tosone, C., Nuttman-Shwartz, O., & Stephens, T. (2012). Shared trauma: When the professional is personal. *Clinical Social Work Journal, 40*(2), 231–239. https://doi.org/10.1007/s10615-012-0395-0

Valutis, S., Rubin, D., & Bell, M. (2012). Professional socialization and social work values: Who are we teaching? *Social Work Education: The International Journal, 31*(8), 1046–1057. https://doi.org/10.1080/02615479.2011.610785

Zerubavel, N., & O'Dougherty-Wright, M. (2012). The dilemma of the wounded healer. *Psychotherapy, 49*(4), 482–491. https://doi.org/10.1037/a0027824

Index

A
Abstinent, 101–103
Acculturative stress, 124

B
Benish-Weisman study, 124
Bereavement, 143, 144, 151
Brenda clinical case, 105–110

C
Childhood sexual trauma, 99
Claustrophobic, 118
Clinicians, 98, 131
Colleen case (spirituality), 79–81
Complex trauma, 44, 53–55
Complicated grief, 144, 150–154
Continuing professional development, 179
The Council on Social Work Education, 175

D
Diagnostic and Statistical Manual of Mental Disorders (DSM-5), 53
Diana's PTSD symptoms, 132–137
Disenfranchised grief, 157

E
Ethnic identity, 117
Ethnicity
  affiliation/disaffiliation, 30
  clients and communities, 26
  and cultural differences, case studies, 33–39
  disenfranchisement, 28
  environmental supports and life skills, 27
  human community, affecting, 20
  identity development, 21, 32
  immigrants, Hispanic, 25, 26
  impressions and assumptions, clients, 31
  jail and prison, theoretical distinction, 22–25
  local communities and neighborhoods, 26
  narrative, 21
  otherness, 22
  in relational context, 21
  social constructions, 20
  socioeconomic factors, 8
  violence, 20

G
Gender
  expectations and cultural scripts, 92
  identity, 100
  sexual orientation, 110
  socioeconomic factors, 8
  stereotypes, 87
  transgender, 86, 87
Grief and loss
  case study, 162–167
  in clinical practice, 161, 162
  description, 143
  dual process model, 145
  Kubler-Ross' framework, 144
  mourning and melancholia, 144
  narratives, 146–150
  physical death, 158–160
  relational track, 145

Grief and loss (*cont.*)
    scriptural texts, religious traditions, 144
    social workers and therapists, 143
    varieties of, 154–158

I

Immigrant
    crafting and re-crafting, 127
    trauma, 129, 130
Immigration
    development of, 113
    and immigrants, 113–114
    journey of, 126
    narrative, 115, 119–124
    phases of, 115, 117, 118
    politics and culture, 130, 131
    process of, 124, 126
    story of, 113
    trauma, 129, 130
    in United States, 114
Institutionalization, 4, 8
Internalized racism, 29
Intimacy, 100, 101
Islamophobia, 74

L

Legitimation, 4
Loss and identity renegotiation, 120, 124

M

Marriage
    description, 4
    as a type, 4
Masturbation, 96
Mature professional identity, 179
Meaningful continuing education, 180
Meaning-making
    systems, 9, 11
    and trauma narrative, 46, 51, 54
Mental illness, 7, 8
Mexican immigrants, 114
Microaggressions, 30
Modernism, 2

N

Narrative, 8–10, 20
    "also true", experience, 12, 13
    with another person, 5
    with Borderline Personality Disorder worker, 10, 11
    at conference, 2
    on countertransference, 6
    to culture
        among adolescents, expressions, 8
        "truth", in psychoanalytic situation, 10
        cognitive and linguistic processes, 10
        grand lives/narratives and "small stories", 10
        meaning-making systems, 9
        mental health and illness, 8
        political polling, 9
        reflexive relationship, 8
        sense of experience, 9
    with depression, struggling, 6
    dominant story lines, 11, 12
    in humility, 4
    as knowers, 3
    marriage, described, 4
    meaning-making, 7
    "narrative turns", 2
    as organic, 13
    postmodernism, 2
    and practice serve, 14
    race, 20 (*see also* Race)
    reality, 2
    reification, process of, 4
    social constructionism, 3
    social constructionist foundations, 7
    in social work practice class/clinical supervision, 5
    story, described, 7
    "storytelling", 13
    temporal and relational, events, 7
    on truth, 3
Narrative turn, 2
Narratives of the professional self, 176
Normal grief, 150–154

O

One drop rule, 21
Otherness, 22, 25, 26, 30

P

Pew Research Center, 114
Philanthropy, 85
Political and cultural rhetoric regarding immigration, 130, 131
Positive and negative spirituality, 67
Positivism, 2
Postmodernism, 2, 3
Posttraumatic growth (PTG), 51
Post-traumatic stress disorder (PTSD), 53–55

Projective identification, 21
Proxemics, 122

R
Race
    affiliation/disaffiliation, 30
    clients and communities, 26
    cumulative advantage, 27
    definition, 21 (*see also* Ethnicity)
    experience, dimension of, 32
    human community, affecting, 20
    impressions and assumptions, clients, 31
    for individuals, 21
    intersectionality, 27
    microaggression, 30
    narrative, 21
    as "one drop rule", 21
    opportunity structures, 27
    in relational context, 21
    social constructions, 20
    on socially constructed forces, 28
    for social work practice and to justice, 22
    socioeconomic factors, 8
    supervision training course, 31
    theoretical distinction, jail and prison, 22–25
    violence, 20
    white privilege, 29
    within-group manifestations, 29
Reality, 2, 4
Reification process, 4
Religious beliefs, 69, 78

S
Sexual development, 86, 87
Sexual identity, 85, 86, 90
Sexual orientation
    client, 90
    genders, 97
    gender expression, 105
    gender identity, 100
    health care, 110
    sexual orientation, 105
    socioeconomic factors, 8
Sexual story
    client's, 87
    sexuality, 86
Sexuality
    area of, 86, 110
    Brenda's sexuality, 108
    client's heterosexuality, 90
    description, 85
    dimensions, 105
    experience of, 106
    genital, 95–100
    human, 86
    individual, 87
    matters of sex, 89
    sense of sex, 91
    and sexual behavior, 90, 95
    and sexual experience, 90
    and sexual story, 88
Social constructionism, 3
Social work, 138
    identity, 174–179
    school, 91
    workers, 131
Spiritual autobiography, 81
Spiritual narrative, 67–71, 74, 75, 77, 78, 82
Spirituality
    children, 70
    clinicians, 69
    description, 67
    individual, communal and social, 71–77
    neurosurgery and orthopedics unit, 70
    people, 68
    and religion, 68
    and religious experience, 67
    social worker, 77–79
    "spiritual but not religious", 68, 69
    spiritual narrative, 68
    students, 70
    US adults, 69
    yoga studios, 68
Storied nature of human conduct, 7

T
Trauma narrative
    approaches, 56–60
    assumptions, 46
    awareness of suicide, 60
    benefit-finding and -reminding, 51
    as broken narrative, 45
    complex trauma, 44, 53–55
    depression, case studies, 60–62
    description, 43
    desire, individuals, 47
    as global and situational meaning, 52
    gun-control debates, 56
    about grief, 59, 60
    impact of loss, 56
    individual experience, 44
    individual traumas, 55

Trauma narrative (*cont.*)
   loss, and suffering, 46
   micro- and macro-narrative, 52
   and meaning making, 46, 51, 54
   and narrative memory, 45
   openness, strategy of, 58
   peace and integration, 50
   perceived self-preservation, 54
   predisposing factors, 44
   principalle strategies, 47
   psychoeducation, 49
   PTG, 51
   PTSD, 53–55
   risk-taking behaviors, 54
   safety and support, 48, 49
   stable and authentic narratives, 45
   9/11, traumatic event, 46, 51
   unspeakable horrors, 55
   in wake of trauma, 51
   wound, 43
Typification, 4

U
Ultimate meaning, 67, 81
The United Nations High Commission on Refugees (UNHCR), 114

V
Victimization, 125

W
White privilege, 29, 30
Wounded healer, 173

CPSIA information can be obtained
at www.ICGtesting.com
Printed in the USA
BVHW01*0718180118
505652BV00007B/25/P